Register Now for Online Access to Your Book!

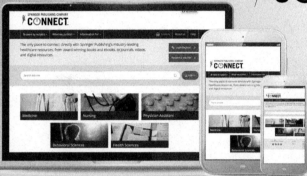

Your print purchase of *McLean EMG Guide, Second Edition* **includes online access to the contents of your book**—increasing accessibility, portability, and searchability!

Access today at:
http://connect.springerpub.com/content/book/978-0-8261-7213-6
or scan the QR code at the right with your smartphone
and enter the access code below.

1JLWU1HY

Scan here for quick access.

If you are experiencing problems accessing the digital component of this product, please contact our customer service department at cs@springerpub.com

The online access with your print purchase is available at the publisher's discretion and may be removed at any time without notice.

Publisher's Note: New and used products purchased from third-party sellers are not guaranteed for quality, authenticity, or access to any included digital components.

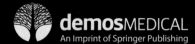

View all our products at springerpub.com/demosmedical

- Femoral mono N — sartorius
- L5 rad vs common fib —
- TOS n — thumb abd, sensory — ulnar / MABC
  C8-T1
- Fem N vs L3 rad — Add long
- Hypothyroidism — distal ① weaker, delayed relaxation of DTR, cramps ②
- CIM — Axonal sensory-motor
  alcohol
  DM —

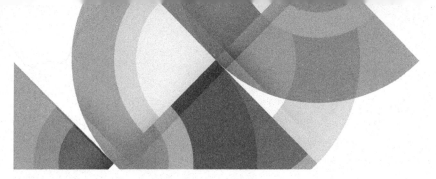

McLean EMG Guide

Second Edition

Editors

Samuel K. Chu, MD
Assistant Professor
Northwestern Feinberg School of Medicine
Attending Physician
Shirley Ryan AbilityLab
Chicago, Illinois

Prakash Jayabalan, MD, PhD
Assistant Professor
Northwestern Feinberg School of Medicine
Attending Physician Scientist
Shirley Ryan AbilityLab
Chicago, Illinois

Christopher J. Visco, MD
Ursula Corning Associate Professor
Sports Medicine Fellowship Director
Residency Program Director
Vice-Chair of Education
Department of Rehabilitation and Regenerative Medicine
Columbia University College of Physicians and Surgeons
New York-Presbyterian Hospital
New York, New York

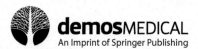

Visit www.springerpub.com and http://connect.springerpub.com

ISBN: 978-0-8261-7212-9
ebook ISBN: 978-0-8261-7213-6
DOI: 10.1891/9780826172136

Acquisitions Editor: Beth Barry
Compositor: S4Carlisle Publishing Services

Copyright © 2019 Springer Publishing Company.

Demos Medical Publishing is an imprint of Springer Publishing Company, LLC.

All rights reserved. This book is protected by copyright. No part of it may be reproduced, stored in a retrieval system, or transmitted in any form or by any means, electronic, mechanical, photocopying, recording, or otherwise, without the prior written permission of the publisher.

Medicine is an ever-changing science. Research and clinical experience are continually expanding our knowledge, in particular our understanding of proper treatment and drug therapy. The authors, editors, and publisher have made every effort to ensure that all information in this book is in accordance with the state of knowledge at the time of production of the book. Nevertheless, the authors, editors, and publisher are not responsible for errors or omissions or for any consequences from application of the information in this book and make no warranty, expressed or implied, with respect to the contents of the publication. Every reader should examine carefully the package inserts accompanying each drug and should carefully check whether the dosage schedules mentioned therein or the contraindications stated by the manufacturer differ from the statements made in this book. Such examination is particularly important with drugs that are either rarely used or have been newly released on the market.

Library of Congress Cataloging-in-Publication Data

Names: Chu, Samuel K., editor. | Jayabalan, Prakash, editor. | Visco, Christopher J., editor.
Title: McLean EMG guide / [edited by] Samuel K. Chu, Prakash Jayabalan, Christopher J. Visco.
Other titles: McLean course in electrodiagnostic medicine | EMG guide
Description: Second edition. | New York : Demos Medical, [2019] | Preceded by McLean course in electrodiagnostic medicine / [edited by] Christopher J. Visco, Gary P. Chimes. c2011. | Includes bibliographical references and index.
Identifiers: LCCN 2019002642 (print) | LCCN 2019003919 (ebook) | ISBN 9780826172136 | ISBN 9780826172129 (alk. paper) | ISBN 9780826172136 (ebook)
Subjects: | MESH: Electrodiagnosis–methods | Neuromuscular Diseases–diagnosis
Classification: LCC RC77 (ebook) | LCC RC77 (print) | NLM WB 141 | DDC 616.07/547–dc23
LC record available at https://lccn.loc.gov/2019002642

Contact us to receive discount rates on bulk purchases.
We can also customize our books to meet your needs.
For more information please contact: sales@springerpub.com

Publisher's Note: New and used products purchased from third-party sellers are not guaranteed for quality, authenticity, or access to any included digital components.

Printed in the United States of America.
19 20 21 22 23 / 5 4 3 2 1

*This book is dedicated to Jim,
may his memory live on.*

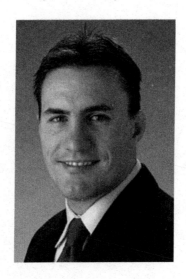

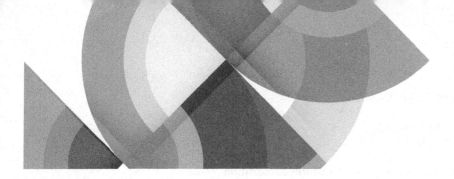

Contents

Contributors xi
Preface xvii

SECTION I. INTRODUCTION

1. Introduction to Electrodiagnostics 3
   Gautam Malhotra

2. Instrumentation 9
   Gautam Malhotra

3. Systematic Approach to Learning and Performing Nerve Conduction Studies 13
   Gautam Malhotra, Jason Bitterman, and Chae K. Im

SECTION II. NERVE CONDUCTION STUDIES

4. Upper Limb Motor Studies 23
   Matthew C. Oswald and Khushboo Doshi

5. Upper Limb Sensory Studies 29
   Byron J. Schneider and David J. Kennedy

6. Lower Limb Motor Studies 37
   Berdale Colorado

7. Lower Limb Sensory Studies 41
   Jacqueline Neal and Nida Gleveckas-Martens

8. F-Waves 55
   Solomon Rojhani and Akhil Chhatre

9. H-Reflexes 61
   Leslie Rydberg

SECTION III. NEEDLE EMG

10. Basic EMG Technique   67
    Christian M. Custodio

11. Basic Approach to EMG Waveform Recognition   73
    Gautam Malhotra and Chae K. Im

12. Motor Unit Action Potential Analysis   81
    Anirudh Gupta, Kasser Saba, and W. David Arnold

13. Recruitment   87
    Monal Desai and W. David Arnold

SECTION IV. IMPORTANT CONCEPTS FOR INTERPRETING STUDIES

14. Orthodromic and Antidromic Nerve Conduction Studies   97
    Daniel A. Goodman

15. Temporal Dispersion and Phase Cancellation   101
    Mary Ann Miknevich and Jenna Meriggi

16. Interpreting Studies   107
    Joelle Gabet and Wendy M. Helkowski

17. Common Anomalies   115
    Nabela Enam and Nigel Shenoy

SECTION V. COMMON CLINICAL ENTITIES

18. Carpal Tunnel Syndrome   127
    Leslie Rydberg

19. Ulnar Neuropathy at the Elbow   135
    Akinpelumi Beckley and Susie S. Kwon

20. Radial Neuropathy   143
    Jonathan S. Kirschner and Carlo Milani

21. Anterior Interosseous Nerve Lesions   153
    Patrick J. Barrett

22. Fibular (Peroneal) Neuropathy   159
    Rohini Sweta Rao and Aaron Jay Yang

23. Tibial Neuropathy   169
    Brian F. White

24. Femoral Neuropathy   177
    Dan Cushman

25. Lumbosacral Radiculopathy   185
    Nathan P. Olafsen and Daniel T. Probst

26. Cervical Radiculopathy   195
    Ryan Doyel and Monica E. Rho

27. Facial Nerve and Blink Studies   203
    Kevin Carneiro and William Filer

28. Repetitive Stimulation and Neuromuscular Junction Disorders   211
    Trevor Gessel and Nassim Rad

29. Peripheral Neuropathy   217
    Michael Mallow

30. Brachial Plexopathy   221
    Christopher J. Visco and Idris Amin

31. Motor Neuron Disease   231
    Dena Abdelshahed, Ankita Dutta, Chae K. Im, and James F. Wyss

32. Myopathy   239
    Gautam Malhotra

33. The Use of Ultrasound With Electrodiagnosis   245
    Jeffrey A. Strakowski

SECTION VI. CHECKLISTS AND ANSWERS

34. Checklists   255

35. Answers to Multiple-Choice Questions   263

Index   281

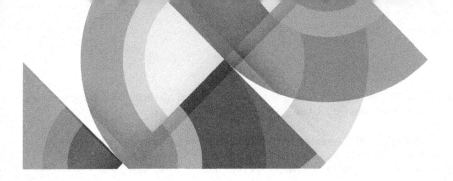

Contributors

Dena Abdelshahed, MD Assistant Attending Physiatrist, Hospital for Special Surgery; Assistant Professor of Rehabilitation Medicine, Department of Physiatry, Weill Cornell Medical College, New York, New York

Idris Amin, MD, CAQSM, FAAPMR Assistant Professor, Sports Medicine Physiatrist, Department of Orthopaedics, University of Maryland, College Park, Maryland

W. David Arnold, MD Associate Professor, Division of Neuromuscular Diseases, Department of Neurology, Department of Physical Medicine and Rehabilitation, Department of Neuroscience, Department of Physiology and Cell Biology, The Ohio State University Wexner Medical Center, Columbus, Ohio

Patrick J. Barrett, MD Assistant Chief, Physical Medicine and Rehabilitation Service, Jesse Brown VA Medical Center; Assistant Professor, Department of Physical Medicine and Rehabilitation, Feinberg School of Medicine, Northwestern University, Chicago, Illinois

Akinpelumi Beckley, MD Assistant Professor, Department of Rehabilitation and Regenerative Medicine, Columbia University Medical Center/New York-Presbyterian Hospital, New York, New York

Jason Bitterman, MD Resident, Department of Physical Medicine and Rehabilitation, Rutgers New Jersey Medical School, Newark, New Jersey; Kessler Institute for Rehabilitation, West Orange, New Jersey

Kevin Carneiro, DO Assistant Professor, Department of Neurosurgery, UNC School of Medicine, Chapel Hill, North Carolina

Akhil Chhatre, MD Director of Spine Rehabilitation; Fellowship Director of Interventional Spine, Sports, and Musculoskeletal Medicine; Assistant Professor, Physical Medicine and Rehabilitation, Johns Hopkins University School of Medicine, Baltimore, Maryland

Berdale Colorado, DO, MPH Assistant Professor, EMG Medical Director, Department of Orthopaedic Surgery, Washington University School of Medicine, St. Louis, Missouri

Dan Cushman, MD Assistant Professor, Division of Physical Medicine and Rehabilitation, University of Utah, Salt Lake City, Utah

Christian M. Custodio, MD Associate Attending Physiatrist, Department of Neurology, Memorial Sloan Kettering Cancer Center; Associate Clinical Professor, Department of Rehabilitation Medicine, Weill Cornell Medical College, New York, New York

Monal Desai, MD Clinical Instructor House Staff, Department of Physical Medicine and Rehabilitation, The Ohio State University Wexner Medical Center, Columbus, Ohio

Khushboo Doshi, MD Resident Physician, Physical Medicine and Rehabilitation, McGaw Graduate Medical Center of Northwestern University–Shirley Ryan AbilityLab, Chicago, Illinois

Ryan Doyel, MD Resident Physician, Department of Physical Medicine and Rehabilitation, Shirley Ryan AbilityLab/Northwestern University, Chicago, Illinois

Ankita Dutta, BA Doctoral Candidate, Icahn School of Medicine at Mount Sinai, CUNY Graduate Center, New York, New York

Nabela Enam, MD Resident Physician, Department of Physical Medicine and Rehabilitation, Rutgers New Jersey Medical School, Newark, New Jersey; Kessler Institute for Rehabilitation, West Orange, New Jersey

William Filer, MD Assistant Professor, Department of Physical Medicine and Rehabilitation, UNC School of Medicine, Chapel Hill, North Carolina

Joelle Gabet, MD PGY-3 Resident, Department of Physical Medicine and Rehabilitation, University of Pittsburgh Medical Center, Pittsburgh, Pennsylvania

Trevor Gessel, MD Fellow, Department of Rehabilitation Medicine, University of Washington, Seattle, Washington

Nida Gleveckas-Martens, DO, MS Assistant Professor, Director, Neurophysiology Laboratory, Department of Neurology, Northwestern University Feinberg School of Medicine; Attending Physician, Neurology, Jesse Brown VA Medical Center, Chicago, Illinois

Daniel A. Goodman, MD, MS Attending Physician, Shirley Ryan AbilityLab; Assistant Professor, Northwestern University Feinberg School of Medicine, Chicago, Illinois

Anirudh Gupta, MD, PhD Clinical Instructor House Staff, Department of Neurology, The Ohio State University Wexner Medical Center, Columbus, Ohio

Wendy M. Helkowski, MD Associate Professor, University of Pittsburgh School of Medicine; Vice-Chair and Residency Program Director, Department of Physical Medicine and Rehabilitation, University of Pittsburgh Medical Center, Pittsburgh, Pennsylvania

Chae K. Im, MD Service Chief, Physical Medicine and Rehabilitation Service, VA New Jersey Health Care System, East Orange, New Jersey; Assistant Professor, Department of Physical Medicine and Rehabilitation, Rutgers New Jersey Medical School, Newark, New Jersey

David J. Kennedy, MD Professor and Chair, Department of Physical Medicine and Rehabilitation, Vanderbilt University Medical Center, Nashville, Tennessee

Jonathan S. Kirschner, MD Physiatry Fellowship Director, Interventional Spine and Sports Medicine, Associate Attending Physiatrist, Department of Physiatry, Hospital for Special Surgery; Associate Professor of Clinical Rehabilitation Medicine, Department of Rehabilitation Medicine, Weill Cornell Medicine, New York, New York

Susie S. Kwon, MD Resident, Department of Rehabilitation Medicine, New York-Presbyterian Hospital, New York, New York

Gautam Malhotra, MD Attending Physician, Physical Medicine and Rehabilitation Service, VA New Jersey Health Care System, East Orange, New Jersey; Associate Professor, Department of Physical Medicine and Rehabilitation, Rutgers New Jersey Medical School, Newark, New Jersey

Michael Mallow, MD Assistant Professor, Residency Program Director, Department of Rehabilitation Medicine, Sidney Kimmel Medical College at Thomas Jefferson University, Philadelphia, Pennsylvania

Jenna Meriggi, DO PGY-3 Resident, Department of Physical Medicine and Rehabilitation, University of Pittsburgh Medical Center, Pittsburgh, Pennsylvania

Mary Ann Miknevich, MD Clinical Assistant Professor, University of Pittsburgh School of Medicine; Associate Residency Director, Department of Physical Medicine and Rehabilitation, University of Pittsburgh Medical Center, Pittsburgh, Pennsylvania

Carlo Milani, MD, MBA Assistant Attending Physiatrist, Department of Physiatry, Hospital for Special Surgery; Assistant Professor of Clinical Rehabilitation Medicine, Department of Rehabilitation Medicine, Weill Cornell Medicine, New York, New York

Jacqueline Neal, MD, MSE Assistant Professor, Department of Physical Medicine and Rehabilitation, Northwestern University Feinberg School of Medicine; Attending Physician, Physical Medicine and Rehabilitation, Jesse Brown VA Medical Center, Chicago, Illinois

Nathan P. Olafsen, MD Assistant Professor, Division of Physical Medicine and Rehabilitation, Department of Orthopaedic Surgery, Washington University School of Medicine, St. Louis, Missouri

Matthew C. Oswald, MD Assistant Professor, Department of Physical Medicine and Rehabilitation, Northwestern University Feinberg School of Medicine; Attending Physician, Department of Physical Medicine and Rehabilitation, Shirley Ryan AbilityLab, Chicago, Illinois

Daniel T. Probst, MD   Resident Physician, Division of Physical Medicine and Rehabilitation, Department of Neurology, Washington University School of Medicine, St. Louis, Missouri

Nassim Rad, MD   Assistant Professor, Department of Rehabilitation Medicine, University of Washington, Seattle, Washington

Rohini Sweta Rao, MD   Resident Physician, Department of Physical Medicine and Rehabilitation, Vanderbilt University Medical Center, Nashville, Tennessee

Monica E. Rho, MD, MPH   Director of Residency Training, Chief of Musculoskeletal Medicine, Department of Physical Medicine and Rehabilitation, Shirley Ryan AbilityLab/Northwestern University, Chicago, Illinois

Solomon Rojhani, MD   Clinical Instructor, Department of Orthopedic Surgery, University of California, Los Angeles, Los Angeles, California

Leslie Rydberg, MD   Assistant Professor, Department of Physical Medicine and Rehabilitation, Northwestern University Feinberg School of Medicine; Attending Physician, Department of Physical Medicine and Rehabilitation, Shirley Ryan AbilityLab, Chicago, Illinois

Kasser Saba, MD   Clinical Instructor House Staff, Department of Neurology, The Ohio State University Wexner Medical Center, Columbus, Ohio

Byron J. Schneider, MD   Assistant Professor, Department of Physical Medicine and Rehabilitation, Vanderbilt University Medical Center, Nashville, Tennessee

Nigel Shenoy, MD   Assistant Chief, Department of Physical Medicine and Rehabilitation, VA New Jersey Health Care System; Clinical Assistant Professor, Department of Physical Medicine and Rehabilitation, Rutgers New Jersey Medical School, Newark, New Jersey

Jeffrey A. Strakowski, MD   Associate Director, Riverside Methodist Hospital, Department of Physical Medicine and Rehabilitation, The Ohio State University, Columbus, Ohio

Christopher J. Visco, MD   Ursula Corning Associate Professor, Sports Medicine Fellowship Director, Residency Program Director, Vice-Chair of Education, Department of Rehabilitation and Regenerative Medicine, Columbia University College of Physicians and Surgeons, New York-Presbyterian Hospital, New York, New York

Brian F. White, DO   Attending Physician, Interventional Pain and Electrodiagnostics, Department of Surgery, Bassett Healthcare, Cooperstown, New York

James F. Wyss, MD, PT   Assistant Attending Physiatrist, Associate Fellowship Director, Director of Education for HSS Physiatry Department, Hospital for Special Surgery; Assistant Professor of Rehabilitation Medicine, Department of Physiatry, Weill Cornell Medical College, New York, New York

Aaron Jay Yang, MD   Assistant Professor, Department of Physical Medicine and Rehabilitation, Vanderbilt University Medical Center, Nashville, Tennessee

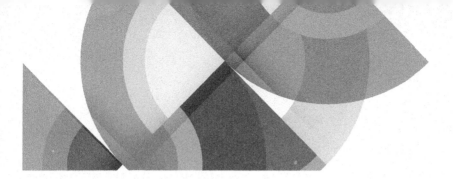

Preface

As junior residents trying to learn about electrodiagnostic medicine, we went into rotations with some trepidation, overwhelmed by both the amount and the type of practical learning required to be a successful electrodiagnostician. We looked for a text that could provide the basics, including EMG and nerve conduction study terminology and definitions, the practicalities of the setup for studies, as well as clinical pearls and troubleshooting. Then, we found the *McLean Course in Electrodiagnostic Medicine*, First Edition. This book transformed how we thought about EMG—suddenly everything seemed less daunting and learning became more enjoyable and streamlined. The original book provided us with a practical and concise text for our EMG rotations and was a great companion to the larger reference texts that successful electrodiagnosticians also need.

We are now honored to be a part of updating the original edition. The new text we are providing here includes more of the practical information on EMGs that made the first edition so successful and we have changed the title to *McLean EMG Guide* to reflect this emphasis. In addition, we have updated the pictures, text, clinical pearls, questions, and tables and provided novel chapters, such as the use of ultrasound in electrodiagnostics. These chapters are written by some of the foremost and experienced authorities in the field.

We want to acknowledge and thank the original editors of this text, Chris Visco and Gary Chimes, who had the incredible vision to create a text that is ideal for both trainees starting out and the electrodiagnostician who needs background, pearls, and practical information. This new edition also continues the legacy of Dr. Jim McLean, who was the inspiration behind the original text. Jim had been a resident at Kessler and then a sports medicine fellow at the Rehabilitation Institute of Chicago (RIC). We followed in the footsteps of Jim as sports medicine fellows at RIC, and we remember our mentors during fellowship, including Dr. Joel Press, always speaking so fondly of Jim and particularly of his gift of being a fantastic teacher. Teaching was clearly a passion of Jim's, and he left a lasting impression on his trainees, who continue to pay forward the time he dedicated to the pursuit of educational excellence.

Samuel K. Chu
Prakash Jayabalan

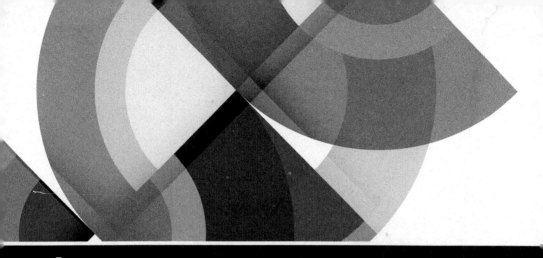

I INTRODUCTION

[Brachial plexus]
(15 nerves)

```
     1'    0     1    3
    Cord  Div  Trunk Root
                     DNL-1,2,3
```

- Musculocutaneous
- Axillary
- Median
- Radial
- Ulnar

lat. pectoral   subscap.2

TARUL
LPR

MC   MC
forearm arm

- C5
- C6
- C7
- C8
- T1

Med wig bgy thru
lat. accy

Lumbosacral
D1 - large abd
   Mcv cf flx

[Lumbar plexus]
(8 nerves)

1 iliohypogastric
1 ilioinguinal
2 Genitofemoral
2,3 LFCN
2,3,4 Femoral
2,3,4 Obturator

- L1
- L2
- L3
- L4
- L5

accessory
obturator 3,4

Lumbosacral
trunk   4,5

[Sacral plexus] (3 or up to)
(5 nerves)

G med, G min, TFL   SG L4 L5 S1
G max   IG up to L5 S1 S2
                     Sciatic fibular - up to S2
                             Tibial - up to S3
                     Post. fem S1 S2 S3
                     Pudendal   S2 S3 S4

- L4   TA - DF, i
- L5   PT - PF, e
- S1   PB - PF, e
- S2
- S3
- S4

Ach reflex - S1
Pat reflex - L4
Meo

EPB ECRB   EPL EDS EPM EC
APL ECRL   SIP

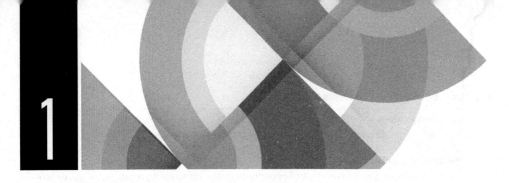

Introduction to Electrodiagnostics

Gautam Malhotra

BASIC PRINCIPLES OF ELECTRODIAGNOSTICS

- The human body constantly generates electrical energy. Specifically, the muscle and nerve cells constantly use electric discharges to communicate among different parts of the body.
- These electric discharges can be recorded, displayed, measured, and interpreted by using specialized equipment.
- In the presence of disease or injury, the architecture and normal processes of nerves and muscles are altered. Recognizing these changes can be useful for diagnosis, monitoring disease progression, and assessing treatments.
- **Electrodiagnostic (EDX)** medicine is the process of observing and interpreting neuromuscular electrical discharges for clinical purposes. We use "EDX" for the remainder of this book to represent this testing, which includes **nerve conduction studies (NCS)** and **electromyography (EMG)**.

BASIC LOGISTICAL DETAILS FOR YOUR FIRST DAY PERFORMING ELECTRODIAGNOSTICS

- The novice EDX consultant (from here on referred to as "you") is faced with learning many new concepts in parallel and at once.
- These include the associated basic science concepts (Table 1.1), hands-on EDX procedures, and analysis of the EDX results. The second basic concept—the hands-on EDX procedure—is the emphasis of this book.
- At first, you will just perform the procedures of an algorithm accurately and efficiently under the guidance of your instructor.
- Once your hands are moving easily from one procedure to the next, you should be able to spontaneously analyze on the fly and mentally adjust a dynamic algorithm.

TABLE 1.1 Basic Science Concepts to Learn

Membrane Physiology
• How physiologic discharges are generated by the cell membrane

Volume Conduction Theory
• How electrical discharges spread and propagate in any conducting medium as governed by the laws of physics

Neuromuscular Physiology
• Structures and functions of the motor unit, sensory nerve, and associated connective tissue

Body's Response to Injury
• Morphologic and electrical timing and changes associated with different types of injury (e.g., demyelination vs. axonal damage)

Anatomic Innervations
• Dermatomes and myotomes at the level of the root, plexus, and peripheral nerve

BASIC CONSTRUCTION OF AN ELECTRODIAGNOSTIC CONSULT

Consult Request

- You will be consulted by a clinician who will send all types of chief complaints to "rule out" things. These usually include complaints of numbness, tingling, or weakness. You should view the referral simply as a guideline or starting point for the EDX visit.
- The EDX encounter is different from a regular consult because the emphasis is placed on you as a technician. Therefore, you may want to be more focused and direct without sacrificing professionalism, compassion, or congeniality. Look for possible contraindications (see Box 3.3 in Chapter 3) prior to performing the procedure. Point out reasonable expectations of the test to your patients and warn them that it is uncomfortable but well tolerated by most people.

History

- This is the time to establish a broad differential diagnosis. Try to figure out which body system is involved. Is the etiology neurological? Musculoskeletal? Psychological? Bilateral? Proximal versus distal?

Physical Examination

- At this time, you will essentially confirm your thoughts using the history. This will inform and direct your EDX testing, which should never be set in stone.

Nerve Conduction Studies

- Typically, this is the first part of the EDX examination. You will stimulate nerves by delivering an electrical current usually via a stimulator wand. The axons of the stimulated nerve generate action potentials that propagate both proximally and distally from the site of stimulation. Electrodes placed over the nerve or a relevant muscle "pick up" the action potential as it propagates under them. The electrical **signal** that is picked up by the electrodes is amplified, filtered, and processed by the equipment.

Motor unit amplitude - monopolar - 1-7 mV

Introduction to Electrodiagnostics | 5

- The signal is converted to a **waveform** (aka *evoked response*) that is displayed on a screen. The x-axis represents time (usually in milliseconds) and the y-axis represents voltage (millivolts or microvolts). Considering units of measure is *very* important prior to analysis of the waveform. Properties of the nerves and muscles can be extrapolated and analyzed thereafter. Certain changes in specific attributes of the waveform can reveal the presence or absence of pathology.

Sensory Nerve Conduction Studies

- Pick-up electrodes are placed over sensory nerves. Stimulation of the corresponding nerve (typically proximally) results in a **sensory nerve action potential** (aka SNAP) on the screen. The SNAP is the electrical signal summation of discharges by the sensory neuron's depolarizing membranes (i.e., axolemma) beneath the pick-up electrodes (Table 1.2).

TABLE 1.2 Features of the Evoked Response

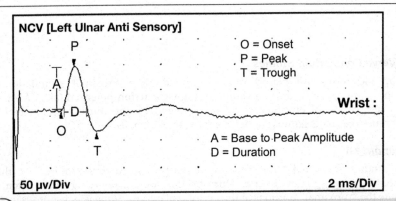

Latency
- *Latency* is the time between the stimulus and the response. In motor nerve studies, latency includes the nerve conduction time and also the neuromuscular transmission time
- Onset latency: Time from stimulation to initial deflection from baseline
- Peak latency: Time from stimulation to upward peak

Amplitude
- The amplitude is dependent on the number of axons that conduct impulses from the stimulus point to the muscle, the number of functioning motor endplates, and the muscle volume.
- The amplitude is measured from the baseline to the upward peak (base-to-peak) or from the upward to downward peak (peak-to-peak).

(continued)

TABLE 1.2 Features of the Evoked Response (*continued*)

Duration
- The duration reflects the synchrony of individual muscle fiber discharges. If there is a significant difference in the conduction velocity among nerve fibers, the duration will be prolonged. This is mainly related to the range of the conduction velocities of the large myelinated fibers.
- Duration is measured from the onset to the first negative to positive baseline crossing.
- Rise time: This is the duration from onset to peak latencies.

Area
- *Area* refers to the integrated area between the compound muscle action potential and the baseline.
- The area represents a combination of the amplitude and the duration. It therefore reflects the number and synchrony of the muscle fibers activated.
- A prolongation of the duration can cause a decrease in the amplitude and may be misinterpreted as a conduction problem. In this situation, there may not be significant difference in the area.

Motor Nerve Conduction Studies

- Pick-up electrodes are placed over a muscle belly. Proximal stimulation of the corresponding nerve produces a **compound muscle action potential** (aka *CMAP*), which is the summation of electrical signals discharged by the muscle fibers' depolarizing membranes (i.e., sarcolemma) under the pick-up electrodes.

Late Responses

- These studies are called "late" because of the prolonged time required for the distal stimulus to travel proximally and return back to the periphery. They are often used to evaluate the *proximal* portions of the peripheral nerves. Some late responses include the H-reflex, F-wave, and A-wave.

Evoked Potentials

- Stimulation occurs at the periphery and pick-up electrodes are placed proximally over the scalp and other areas. Sometimes they are used intraoperatively for monitoring. These include:
  - Auditory-evoked potentials, usually recorded from the scalp but originating at the brainstem level (auditory brainstem response, brainstem auditory-evoked response, brainstem-evoked response, brainstem-evoked potential [BSEP])
  - Visual-evoked potentials
  - Somatosensory-evoked potentials — dorsal column
  - Peripheral sensory nerve stimulation
  - Motor-evoked potentials
  - Peripheral motor nerve stimulation

Electromyography

Typically, this is the last part of the EDX evaluation. A needle electrode is inserted through the skin and fascia to penetrate into the muscle and irritate its membrane (the *sarcolemma*). This irritation elicits transient discharges from the sarcolemma that are picked up by the needle electrode and displayed as waveforms. These waveforms are then analyzed by you (the person performing the test, the EDX consultant). Voluntary and spontaneous electrical discharges by the sarcolemma can be detected by the needle electrode and observed on a screen.

Involuntary Attributes
- Insertional activity: Bursts of electrical discharge directly correlated with irritation by the needle electrode
- Normal and abnormal spontaneous discharges (e.g., endplate spikes, positive sharp waves, fibrillation potentials, fasciculation potentials, complex repetitive discharges, myotonic discharges, myokymic discharges, etc.)

Voluntary Attributes
- Motor unit action potential (MUAP) morphology
- MUAP activation
- MUAP recruitment

EXPLANATION OF FINDINGS

Although the final report will not yet be complete, preliminary findings should be discussed with the patient after the encounter.

ADDITIONAL READINGS

Dumitru D, Amato AA, Zwarts MJ. *Electrodiagnostic Medicine*. 2002.
Wilbourn AJ. Nerve conduction studies. Types, components, abnormalities, and value in localization. *Neurol Clin*. 2002;20(2):305–338, v.

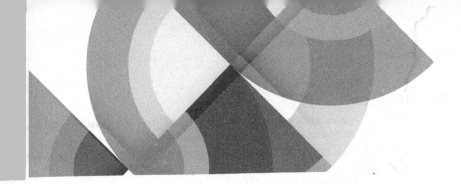

Instrumentation

Gautam Malhotra

INTRODUCTION

Just like any other piece of machinery, your electrodiagnostic (EDX) equipment can be a source of great frustration. Technical limitations and equipment factors can alter and distort the desired physiologic waveforms. These technically derived distortions can easily be confused with findings seen with disease or injury. The EDX consultant must be aware of these sources of error and learn techniques to minimize them.

Understanding how the electrophysiologic instrument processes and displays biologic signals will help you to avoid misinterpreting erroneously derived data from instrumentation errors. EDX instrumentation is not a "black box," but can be thought of as physical links in a chain, or functionally, like a sequence of events. In this chapter, we acquaint you with the signal path and the nature of the components. A simple but practical description of the inner workings of EDX instrumentation is explained. Refer to Figure 2.1 as you read through the descriptions of the componentry to better visualize their effect on the waveform.

THE ELECTRODES

- The electrode is a small piece of metal that is placed on (surface) or in (needle) the part of the body being studied.
  - All nearby potentials affect the electrode. These potentials not only include those generated by nearby muscles and nerves, but also all other electrical sources such as room lights, electrical machinery, radios, pacemakers, and so on.
  - The electrode is not selective. Its purpose is simply to make contact with the body and conduct the sum of these nearby potentials to the next link in the chain. This summation is called a **signal**.
  - A second electrode is located nearby. It undergoes the same process described for the first electrode; however, because it is in a different location, it will pick up a different signal.
  - Often these electrodes are referred to as E1 and E2 or "active" and "reference." Both electrodes participate in the process.

THE SIGNALS

- Initially, the signals are very small in magnitude. The information in these signals is difficult to measure and interpret in this diminutive state.
  - The signals are transmitted from the two electrodes via cables into **amplifiers** (Figure 2.1).
  - Amplifiers are electrical devices that augment or enlarge the signal fed into them by a predetermined factor (the **gain**).
  - A third electrode, termed the **ground electrode**, is also connected to each of the amplifiers and serves as the zero potential value for all recorded potentials.
  - As described earlier, the neurophysiologic signals of interest exist within an environment filled with electrical noise. This sea of noise is several orders of magnitude larger than the signal being studied. An ideal recording would be one in which this unwanted extraneous electrical noise is eliminated while the neurophysiologic signal is selectively amplified.
  - A **differential amplifier** essentially achieves this: The amplified signal from the nearby electrode is subtracted from the amplified signal of the first electrode. If the electrodes are spaced reasonably close to each other, any electrical activity common to both electrodes (e.g., environmental noise) will be eliminated.
- A signal resulting from differential amplification is now large enough to be observed. In an effort to further isolate the desired neurophysiologic signal, **electronic filters** are used next to remove even more unwanted electrical noise.

THE DISPLAYS

- The now amplified and filtered signal is simultaneously sent to two different components.
  - The first is a **speaker**, where the electrical energy is converted to sound energy. This allows the clinician to "hear" the signal; as you perform more studies, you will begin to appreciate the subtle differences in signal sound and their clinical significance.
  - The second component is a **visual display**, where the signal is visually represented as a **waveform**. The type of display depends on whether the equipment being used is analog or digital.

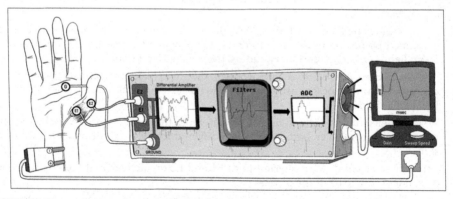

FIGURE 2.1 The author's and artist's playful interpretation of the various physical stages of the electrodiagnostic equipment. Electrodes, attached to the limb, convey the electrical signal through cables into the differential amplifier. The summated signal then passes through filters prior to being sent to a speaker and being converted into a digital signal. This digital signal is then displayed on a screen.

Source: Illustration by Jason Bitterman, MD.

- When older analog-display technology was used, the signal was directly displayed on an oscilloscope screen via a cathode-ray tube. The advantage of this analog display was that a smooth, high-quality continuously varying waveform can be viewed in real time. The major limitation was the difficulty associated with measuring the waveform.
- The newer and now ubiquitous alternative to the analog display is the use of analog-to-digital conversion (ADC). ADC is the conversion of the signal into a numeric format, essentially by a computer. The signal is sampled at discrete time intervals and the amplitude of the signal is converted to a number (digital value). A series of digital values is generated, which provides a close representation of the original analog signal. The advantage of using ADC is that the converted signal can then be stored, manipulated, and examined by digital microprocessors after acquisition. The resultant waveform is then visually displayed on a screen for analysis and interpretation.
- Because the purpose of the test is to measure various parameters, sometimes knobs on the machine can be used to vary the magnification of the displayed signal. Throughout an EDX evaluation, the examiner must maintain constant attention to the units of measurement.
  - The x-axis on the display represents time. The number of seconds (usually milliseconds) measured per division on the screen is known as the **sweep speed**.
  - The y-axis on the display represents voltage. The number of volts (varying from micro- to millivolts) measured per division on the screen is known as the display **sensitivity**.[1]

THE STIMULATOR

- As described earlier, the "pick-up" electrodes are used to detect voltages that are amplified, processed, and displayed. Very often, when performing nerve conduction studies (NCS), neuromuscular measurements require another distinct set of electrodes to deliver an exogenous current.
- The **cathode** is negatively charged (attracts cations) and the **anode** is positively charged (attracting anions). When applied to the surface of the skin, charges flow throughout the body and from one electrode to the other along the paths of least resistance (i.e., the extracellular fluid and skin).
- Current delivered by these **stimulator** (cathode/anode) electrodes is detected by the pick-up electrodes as "stimulus artifact" and treated as time equal to zero.
- If this stimulus current is of sufficient intensity to reach excitable tissues, **action potentials** can be induced to propagate along nerve or muscle membranes.

---

[1] The knob on some machines may be labeled as "gain," which is technically not the same as "sensitivity." *Gain* is the factor by which the input signal is being multiplied within the differential amplifier. *Sensitivity* is the number of units per division displayed on the y-axis. Turning the knob does increase sensitivity and gain staging (per discussion with engineers of electrodiagnostic equipment).

QUESTIONS

1. Which is the correct order of the signal path?
   A. Electrodes → filters → differential amplifier → computer → screen
   B. Electrodes → differential amplifier → ground loop → filters → screen
   C. Electrodes → differential amplifier → filters → computer → screen
   D. Electrodes → signal processor → differential amplifier → filters → computer → screen

2. The signal is sent to the speaker after which of the following components of the signal chain?
   A. Electrodes
   B. Differential amplifier
   C. Filters
   D. Computer

3. Which of the following would be observed if both of the electrodes were placed on exactly the same place on the body?
   A. Flatline
   B. A signal that appears to be twice as large
   C. A signal that appears to be half as large
   D. No difference; interelectrode separation has no effect on the observed waveform

4. Which of the following electrodes is definitively negatively charged?
   A. Anode
   B. Ground
   C. Cathode
   D. Reference

5. Which of the following is a unitless number representing the amount by which an amplifier amplifies?
   A. Sensitivity
   B. Gain
   C. Sweep
   D. Differential equation

Answers to the questions are located in Chapter 35.

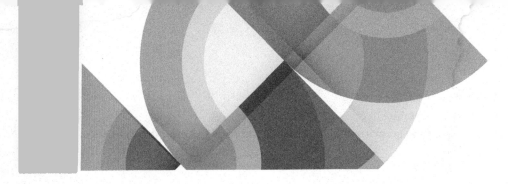

Systematic Approach to Learning and Performing Nerve Conduction Studies

Gautam Malhotra, Jason Bitterman, and Chae K. Im

INTRODUCTION

Electrodiagnostic (EDX) medicine can be intimidating for new learners. This chapter is designed to minimize the discomfort associated with initially performing nerve conduction studies (NCS).

The goal of the protocol described is to provide structure, which should make those first weeks of performing NCS less intimidating. Being systematic in your approach will minimize avoidable inadvertent errors and pitfalls.

The first hurdle in learning NCS is learning the procedure and developing a "muscle memory" so you can later focus on analyzing and managing your studies. If you follow the protocols outlined here, you will learn how to properly prepare and perform an NCS and develop good habits for the future.

This chapter also includes a section on basic troubleshooting for common problems and questions trainees encounter, mainly "Why can't I get my waveform to look right?" Use this section as a starting point whenever you encounter an unusual waveform that you think may be explained by something other than pathology.

NERVE CONDUCTION STUDY CHECKLIST

After performing a focused history, examination, and review of contraindications (see Box 3.3), this checklist should be performed prior to each study and, in particular, before delivering a shock. If done routinely and systematically, the "muscle memory" will take over for future studies and in time the list will become second nature and happen seamlessly. It is important to begin with an environment that is conducive to performing NCS. Whenever possible, this includes a warm, quiet, interference-free environment, which is stocked with the appropriate supplies to limit interruptions.

PRESTUDY CHECKLIST

1. Tape
2. Tape measure
3. Pen
4. Gel

5. Alcohol swabs
6. Check temperature
7. Have access to normal values for latencies and amplitudes for the studies you plan to perform
8. Verbal consent

PRESHOCK CHECKLIST

1. At the patient
   - Make sure that the correct study is being performed.
   - Check the side of the body.
   - Check that stimulation sites have been marked appropriately.
   - Confirm the patient is in proper positioning for the study and the limb is fully exposed.
   - For sensory studies, verify the patient was swabbed with alcohol at the electrode sites.
   - Verify that the ground, active (E1), and reference (E2) electrodes are secured in place.
   - For sensory studies, verify there is at least a 4-cm (upper limb) or 3.2-cm (lower limb) separation between the active and reference electrodes.
2. At the amplifier
   - Verify that the ground, active, and reference electrodes are plugged in.
   - Make sure that they are plugged into the correct channel.
   - Make sure that the amplifier is turned on.
3. At the screen
   - Verify the study on the screen matches that of the patient.
   - Verify the side indicated on the screen matches the side being studied.
   - Check stimulation intensity.
4. At the stimulator
   - Check stimulation intensity, start low.
   - Check cathode and anode position.
5. Shock

SHOCK CHECKLIST

1. Start with a low-intensity stimulation (~10 mA).[1]
2. Increase intensity by about 5 to 10 mA for each subsequent shock until a waveform is visible.

---

[1]There is great variation in opinions on how to begin stimulation. It is the lead author's practice to start at 5 mA on the very first stimulation of the test to acclimate the patient to the discomfort. "It will initially feel like tapping and eventually progress to an electrical shock-like feeling." Some technicians advocate for stimulating at 100 mA from the beginning in an effort to achieve supramaximal stimulation for minimal shocks to the patient; however, this is likely to lead to other problems (see Box 3.2).

3. Once a waveform is visible, ensure that the stimulator is optimally located over the nerve by moving the cathode slightly medially and laterally from your initial shock point looking for the largest possible amplitude.
4. Continue raising stimulation intensity until the waveform's amplitude stops increasing (i.e., *maximal stimulation*). Observe for any dramatic changes in morphology along the way.
5. Add 20% more intensity and shock (i.e., *supramaximal* stimulation).
6. Store the trace.
7. Repeat at the next site.
8. Record measurements between cathode stim points.

Definitions for words used to describe the delivered stimulation current intensities are given in Box 3.1.

BOX 3.1 Stimulation Terminology

> These terms are important for analyzing and troubleshooting your studies. Note that these terms do not describe a numerical intensity but rather how different intensities evoke and affect a waveform.
>
> ### Subthreshold Stimulation
> Stimulation intensities that do not evoke a waveform.
>
> ### Threshold Stimulation
> The minimum amount of stimulation required to visibly evoke a waveform.
>
> ### Submaximal Stimulation
> Any stimulation intensity between threshold and maximal stimulation. In theory, the nerve is not being fully stimulated at this intensity and you are potentially not capturing data for all of the nerve's axons.
>
> ### Maximal Stimulation
> The level of stimulation at which any higher intensity does not increase the waveform amplitude.
>
> ### Supramaximal Stimulation
> Intensity that is approximately 20% greater than maximal stimulation. This is the stimulation level measured for most NCS as it attempts to ensure that all axons within the nerve are stimulated.
>
> ### Overstimulation
> This refers to stimulation beyond the supramaximal intensity (see Box 3.2).

BOX 3.2 The Problems With Overstimulation

Excessive stimulation can cause several erroneous findings that can lead to incorrect analysis of a nerve conduction study. The excessive current flows throughout the body beyond the stimulated nerve. This may result in co-stimulation of nearby nerves.

Any of the following findings may prompt the need to consider overstimulation:

- **Initial positive deflection:** The key finding of overstimulation is an initial positive (downward) deflection rather than an initial negative (upward) deflection. The surface electrode detects an advancing depolarization from nearby co-stimulated nerves, resulting in a positive deflection.
Electrodes record positive deflections from advancing and retreating depolarizations. Electrodes record negative deflections from depolarizations occurring directly below them. Accurate measurement of latency requires an initial negative deflection as that represents detection of depolarization of the tested nerve or muscle directly beneath the active electrode.
- **Increased amplitude:** An artifactually increased amplitude may be detected due to summation of signals from nearby muscles at the distal recording location. Overstimulation often explains larger proximal amplitudes (when you would expect them to be smaller than their distal counterparts).
- **Shortened onset latency:** Excessive current may displace the site of excitation on the nerve up to 12 mm distally from the actual cathode site. This in turn will decrease the amount of time for the current to be recorded distally, resulting in an artifactually shortened onset latency.

BOX 3.3 Risks and Contraindications for NCS[2]

It is essential to know the risks associated with electrodiagnostic testing when assessing subjects for eligibility and for consent.

Intravenous and Central Lines

There is a risk of current from NCS conducting to the heart. As a result, NCS should not be performed in patients with central lines. Peripheral intravenous lines are safe to use assuming there is no fluid running through the line, as the fluid can potentially send current to the heart.

Pacemakers and Defibrillators

Theoretically, stimulation near a cardiac device may achieve a high enough voltage to interfere with the device's programming. In practice, studies have shown that NCS has no effect on internal bipolar pacemakers and defibrillators.

There is at least one reported incident of a unipolar pacemaker being inhibited. Thus, caution is advised for these devices. External pacemakers carry a larger risk of conducting current to the heart and NCS should not be performed.

(*continued*)

---

[2]For more details on risks and contraindications, refer to The American Association of Neuromuscular and Electrodiagnostic Medicine. *Position Statement: Risks of Electrodiagnostic Medicine.* July 2014:1–8. https://www.aanem.org/getmedia/653e87b3-f930-4951-9bd8-dde95c291ce2/risksinEDX.pdf

BOX 3.3 Risks and Contraindications for NCS[2] (*continued*)

Spinal Cord and Deep Brain Stimulators
Theoretically, NCS may influence or interfere with the current in the stimulator leads, resulting in either inhibition or increased stimulation by the stimulator device. Clinicians should weigh the risks and benefits carefully in performing NCS in patients with these devices.

Pregnancy
There is currently no evidence that NCS cause harm in pregnancy. It is to the clinician's discretion to weigh the risks and benefits.

NCS, nerve conduction studies.

REVIEW DURING THE NERVE CONDUCTION STUDIES
Check and Recheck

- Instrument settings
- Electrode placements
- Temperature
- Know your machine setting; that is, peak versus onset latency, or peak-to-peak versus base-to-peak amplitudes

Commit to the Waveform
Prior to storing the evoked waveform, quickly ask yourself whether it makes sense. Do this by looking at the morphology, amplitude, and latency.

- How does this waveform compare with the last one you stored?
- Is it too wide, big, or small compared with what you expected? This could be due to submaximal stimulation, overstimulation, or possibly anomalous innervation.
- Were you able to consistently obtain this waveform or was it the only "lucky" one you got after 20 shocks? Sometimes an artifact looks like it "could be" the correct waveform.
- Ensure that the cursors are in the correct locations. Computers do the best they can at estimating onsets and amplitudes, but *you* are the expert.

Declare an Educated Opinion About the NCS
For example, what do you think of the left median nerve after obtaining compound muscle action potentials (CMAPs) from stimulating at the wrist and elbow? Normal? Abnormal? Borderline? Technically challenging? Your declaration will help to direct which study to do next.

AFTER THE NERVE CONDUCTION STUDIES

Look at Every Value From Every Stimulation and Summarize Them in Written Words

This should be easier to do if you followed the steps outlined earlier. This is an extremely crucial step. Many machines may automatically indicate values that lie outside normal values, but these cannot be relied upon blindly. For example, sometimes the patient's anatomy necessitates stimulation at an atypical distance. The latency and conduction velocity may appear to be abnormal if not taking the new distance into consideration.

Summarize the Entire NCS

This step helps to clarify the differential diagnosis. For example, all lower limb CMAPs were normal and sensory nerve action potentials (SNAPs) were low amplitude, but this could be attributed to the patient's advanced age, extra soft tissue, or edema, and not neuropathic in nature.

Reconcile the Findings With an Exhaustively Comprehensive Neuromuscular Differential Diagnosis

This ensures that a diagnosis is not missed. For example, in establishing carpal tunnel syndrome, an ulnar entrapment or polyneuropathy might be discovered. It also helps to guide the electromyographic testing, which is conventionally performed after NCS. Incorporating this step is a powerful way to advance neuromuscular education in the EDX laboratory.

COMMON NERVE CONDUCTION STUDY TROUBLESHOOTING

Artifact Management in Sensory Studies

SNAPs are very small, on the order of microvolts. If there is enough artifactual current or "background noise" being recorded by the surface electrodes, your SNAPs may be buried within the "noise" despite achieving threshold stimulation.

In order to minimize these artifacts, verify that:

- The skin below both recording electrodes was properly cleaned.
- Enough (but not too much) gel has been applied to each electrode.
- No "bridging" of gel between the active and reference electrodes exists.
- All electrodes are secured to the skin.
- The wiring of the electrodes or stimulator is not crossing one another.
- Proper filter settings are active on your hardware.

In addition, rotating the anode in different directions, while keeping the cathode anchored, may also assist with reducing the contribution from stimulus artifact.

A CMAP Is Being Evoked in a Sensory Study (aka *Motor Artifact*)

Overstimulation during a sensory study can lead to stimulation of motor fibers within a mixed motor sensory nerve. If these motor fibers' signals are recorded at the distal electrodes, the waveform may be altered. Sensory studies at the hand are particularly susceptible to this.

In order to prevent motor artifact:

- Move your recording electrodes away from potential motor points so you are less likely to capture any muscle action potentials.
  - For example, for an ulnar sensory study, move the ring electrode distally down the fifth digit (while attempting to maintain a 4 cm distance between the electrodes).
- Verify that you are not overstimulating the nerve.

The CMAP Waveform Has an Unusual Shape and Low Amplitude

Whenever your CMAP waveform has an unusual morphology or has an unexpectedly decreased amplitude, check the placement of your electrodes.

The active electrode should be above the motor point of the tested muscle. The reference electrode should be on a nearby region that does not have significant muscle-based electrical activity (ideally the tendon or bony attachment of the muscle).

If the active electrode is above the motor point, it will not directly capture the depolarization originating from the motor point as it should. It will instead record the advancing spread of depolarization. This will result in a waveform with an initial positive deflection. The CMAP amplitude will also be reduced.

If the reference electrode is placed over a portion of the muscle, it will capture some of the muscle's electrical activity. The differential amplifier will subtract this activity from the active electrode's data, resulting in a reduced amplitude and possibly an unusual waveform morphology.

The Proximal Stimulation Waveform Has a Larger Amplitude Than the Distal Waveform

When testing multiple sites along a single nerve, you expect the more proximal sites to have the same or lower amplitudes than the distal sites (see Box 3.4). If the proximal site has a larger amplitude, there are three potential causes:

- Overstimulation at the proximal site—Volume conduction has occurred resulting in co-stimulation of adjacent nerves.
- Submaximal stimulation at the distal site—You are not fully stimulating all of the nerve fibers.
- Anomalous innervation—Atypical anatomic variants distally (e.g., an accessory peroneal nerve) can result in distal CMAP amplitudes being falsely decreased (as the conventional distal stimulation site is not properly stimulating the anomalous nerve).

BOX 3.4 A Checklist for Waveform Analysis (Remember the Acronym "MMOAN")

Markers
Are the marker placements for onset latency and peak latency accurate? Do not assume the computer will properly mark latencies.

Morphology
Does the morphology make sense for a CMAP/SNAP?
Are morphologies consistent from one stimulation to the next?

Onset Latency
Is the onset latency within normal limits?

Amplitude
Is the amplitude within normal limits?
  How does the amplitude compare between distal and proximal stimulations?
  - Distal stimulation recordings generally have a larger amplitude than proximal stimulation recordings. This is due to **temporal dispersion and phase cancellation** (see Chapter 17 for more details).

(continued)

BOX 3.4 A Checklist for Waveform Analysis (Remember the Acronym "MMOAN") (*continued*)

- A cause for any significant drop in amplitude from distal to proximal must be explained. In general, for motor studies, the authors suggest 30% on motor studies (with the exception of tibial nerve motor studies, where up to a 50% drop is allowed). Greater than this much is unlikely to be attributable solely to temporal dispersion and phase cancellation. No such cutoff is offered for sensory studies, as they exhibit far more susceptibility to temporal dispersion and phase cancellation with longer distances.

Nerve Conduction Velocity

Is the conduction velocity within normal limits?

- If the conduction velocity for a motor study is abnormal, confirm proper measurement of the distances between stimulation sites.

Is there a difference in conduction velocity between distal and proximal stimulations?

- There should be no difference in velocities.
- However, due to human measurement error and differences in conduction due to temperature, some clinicians allow up to a 20% difference in conduction velocity between segments.

CMAP, compound muscle action potentials; SNAP, sensory nerve action potentials.

CONTINUED LEARNING FOR NERVE CONDUCTION STUDIES

NCSs are a unique procedure. Relatively little dexterity, physical training, or visual–spatial coordination is required to perform an NCS. This is what makes them seem deceivingly easy to perform after initially learning the basics of sticking the electrodes to skin and delivering the shocks.

If this is the end of the learning, the trainee either becomes extremely frustrated or learns to accept a novice level of EDX acumen. It is essential that trainees develop a systematic approach not only to the technical aspects of NCS, but also to the reflection and analysis.

Practicing reflection during and after the study will guarantee the most opportunities for active learning from each NCS encounter. This should always be accompanied by discussion with the mentor followed by reading of the relevant literature.

ADDITIONAL READINGS

American Association of Neuromuscular and Electrodiagnostic Medicine. *Guidelines and Practice Parameters*. http://www.aanem.org/Practice/Practice-FAQs

Dumitru D, Amato AA, Zwarts MJ. *Electrodiagnostic Medicine*. Philadelphia, PA: Hanley & Belfus; 2002.

Gitter AJ, Stolov WC. AAEM minimonograph #16: instrumentation and measurement in electrodiagnostic medicine—Part II. *Muscle Nerve*. 1995;18(8):812-824. doi:10.1002/mus.880180804

Preston DC, Shapiro BE. *Electromyography and Neuromuscular Disorders: Clinical-Electrophysiologic Correlations*. Philadelphia, PA: Butterworth-Heinemann; 2005.

Wilbourn AJ. Nerve conduction studies. Types, components, abnormalities, and value in localization. *Neurol Clin*. 2002;20(2):305–338 PubMed PMID: 12152438.

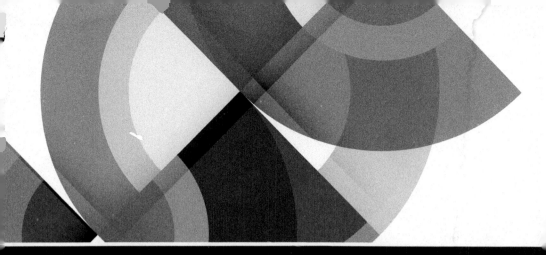

II NERVE CONDUCTION STUDIES

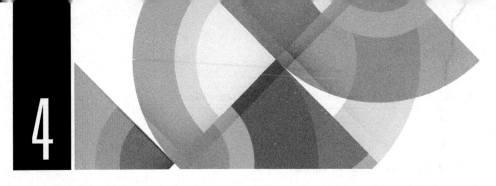

4

Upper Limb Motor Studies

Matthew C. Oswald and Khushboo Doshi

INTRODUCTION

- Motor nerve conduction studies (NCSs) are helpful in the diagnostic assessment of numerous types of pathology, including mononeuropathy, polyneuropathy, plexopathy, and radiculopathy.
- The median and ulnar nerves are the most frequently tested upper limb motor NCSs. Radial motor NCS is performed in select clinical scenarios (Table 4.1).
- Motor NCSs are recorded at a distal muscle innervated by the respective nerve.
- Serial stimulations are performed at select sites from distal to proximal along the anatomic course of the nerve.
- The segments between the stimulation points encompass potential sites of pathology.
- NCS analyze the latency, amplitude, and conduction velocity across each segment in order to identify, localize, and characterize the type of pathology.

TABLE 4.1 Median and Ulnar Muscles of the Hand

Median Muscles of the Hand: A Helpful Reminder Is "LOAF"
Lumbricals (lateral two)
Opponens pollicis
Abductor pollicis brevis
Flexor pollicis brevis (superficial head)
Ulnar Muscles of the Hand: The Ulnar Nerve Also Innervates its Own LOAF Muscles and the Remaining Hand Intrinsics
Lumbricals (Medial two)
Muscles of the hypothenar eminence:
Opponens digiti minimi
Abductor digiti minimi
Flexor digiti minimi

(continued)

TABLE 4.1 Median and Ulnar Muscles of the Hand (*continued*)

Interossei: DABs   PADs
Select muscles of the thenar eminence: Adductor pollicis   Flexor pollicis brevis (deep head)
DABs, dorsal abductors; PADs, palmar adductors.

MEDIAN NERVE

- Recording site:
  - The distal recording site is over the abductor pollicis brevis (APB).
  - The active electrode (E1) is placed over the center of the APB muscle.
  - The reference electrode (E2) is placed over the first metacarpophalangeal joint (MCP).
- Stimulation sites (Table 4.2):
  - S1—Above the wrist, 8 cm proximal to E1 between the flexor carpi radialis and the palmaris longus tendons
  - S2—Elbow: medial to the biceps tendon in the antecubital fossa
- Additional studies include the recurrent branch of the median nerve stimulated in the midpalm. This study evaluates signal amplitude distal to the carpal tunnel. This segment of the nerve is variable in length and course; therefore, the latency and conduction velocity may be unreliable.

ULNAR NERVE

- Recording site:
  - The distal recording site is over the abductor digiti minimi (ADM).
  - The active electrode (E1) is placed over the midmuscle.
  - The reference electrode (E2) is placed over the 5th MCP.
- Stimulation sites:
  - S1—At the wrist, adjacent to the flexor carpi ulnaris (FCU) tendon, 8 cm proximal to E1
  - S2—"Below elbow" approximately 3 to 4 cm distal to the medial epicondyle to ensure that the nerve has exited the cubital tunnel
  - S3—"Above elbow" posterior to the bicep muscle, 10 cm proximal to the "below elbow" site
- The ulnar nerve should be tested with the shoulder abducted 90° and the elbow flexed 90°. This allows assessment of the nerve with as little slack as possible, making distance measurements more accurate.

TABLE 4.2 Upper Limb Motor Tests

Median to the Abductor Pollicis Brevis

Lead Placement
- E1: APB
- E2: First metacarpophalangeal joint

Stimulation

Wrist:
- 8 cm proximal to E1
- Between flexor carpi radialis and palmaris longus tendons

Elbow:
- Medial to biceps tendon in antecubital fossa

Optional midpalm:
- Medial to the thenar eminence

Clinical Correlates for Segments

Across wrist:
- Carpal tunnel syndrome

Elbow to wrist:
- Forearm pathology
- Pronator teres syndrome

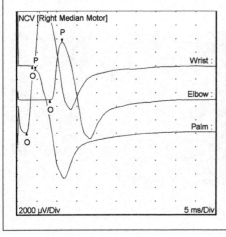
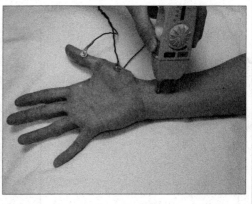

(continued)

RADIAL NERVE

- The radial motor NCS is not routinely assessed. It has diagnostic value when there is clinical weakness or suspicion of radial neuropathy or brachial plexopathy.
- Recording site:
  - The distal recording site is over the extensor indicis proprius (EIP).
  - The active electrode (E1) is placed over the EIP, 4 cm proximal to the ulnar styloid, to ulnar direction of midline.
  - The reference electrode (E2) is placed over the ulnar styloid.

TABLE 4.2 Upper Limb Motor Tests (*continued*)

Ulnar to the Abductor Digiti Minimi	
Lead Placement • E1: ADM • E2: 5th metacarpophalangeal joint	
Stimulation	*Clinical Correlates for Segments*
Wrist: • Medial wrist, adjacent to the FCU tendon (8 cm proximal to E1) Below the elbow: • 3–4 cm distal to the medial epicondyle Above the elbow: • Over the medial humerus, between the biceps and triceps muscles • 10–12 cm from the below-elbow site	Across wrist: • Guyon canal • Below elbow to wrist • Forearm pathology *"Above elbow" to "Below elbow":* • Cubital tunnel syndrome
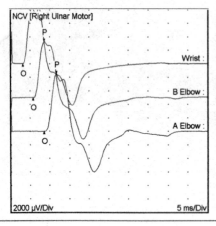	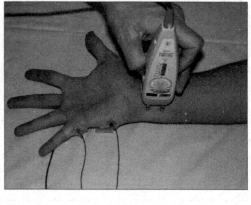

(*continued*)

- Stimulation sites:
  - S1—Forearm: 8 cm proximal to E1 over the dorsal forearm
  - S2—Elbow: Between the biceps and brachioradialis muscles
  - S3—Arm: 8 to 10 cm proximal to the lateral epicondyle, between the biceps and triceps muscles
  - S4—Above the spiral groove: posterior proximal arm

TABLE 4.2 Upper Limb Motor Tests (*continued*)

Radial to the Extensor Indicis Proprius

Lead Placement
- E1: EIP (4 cm proximal to ulnar styloid)
- E2: Ulnar styloid

Stimulation	**Clinical Correlates for Segments**
S1—Forearm:	*Forearm/Elbow to Wrist:*
• 8 cm proximal to EIP	• Dorsal forearm pathology
S2—Elbow:	*Segment S3–S4:*
• In between the biceps and brachioradialis	• Nerve injury at the spiral groove
S3—Arm:	
• 8–10 cm proximal to the lateral epicondyle, between the biceps and triceps	
S4—above spiral groove:	
• Posterior arm against the humerus	

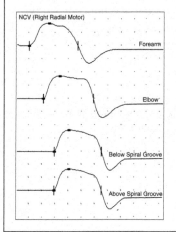
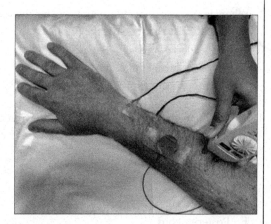

ADM, abductor digiti minimi; APB, abductor pollicis brevis; EIP, extensor indicis proprius; FCU, flexor carpi ulnaris.

NORMAL VALUE RANGE

There are a range of normative values reported in the literature due to differences in technique, patient population, and subject characteristics, including size and age. Therefore, each laboratory should have its own normal values based on the patient population or use a textbook of normal values.

QUESTIONS

1. Which of the following are ulnar-innervated hand muscles?
   A. Adductor pollicis
   B. Abductor digiti minimi
   C. Opponens digiti minimi
   D. Flexor pollicis brevis (deep head)
   E. All of the above

2. In which position should the arm be placed when testing the ulnar motor nerve conduction study?
   A. Arm adducted, elbow extended
   B. Arm abducted, elbow extended
   C. Arm abducted, elbow flexed
   D. Arm adducted, elbow flexed

3. Where is the proximal stimulation site for the median motor nerve conduction study?
   A. At the wrist between the flexor carpi radialis and palmaris longus tendons
   B. At the elbow medial to the biceps tendon
   C. At the elbow lateral to the biceps tendon
   D. In the posterior aspect of the arm

4. The median motor nerve conduction study recorded at abductor pollicis brevis yields diagnostic value for which segments of the brachial plexus (select all)?
   A. Lateral cord
   B. Medial cord
   C. Upper trunk
   D. Lower trunk
   E. Posterior cord

5. The ulnar motor nerve conduction study recorded at abductor digiti minimi yields diagnostic value for which segments of the brachial plexus (select all)?
   A. Lateral cord
   B. Medial cord
   C. Upper trunk
   D. Lower trunk
   E. Posterior cord

Answers to the questions are located in Chapter 35.

5

Upper Limb Sensory Studies

Byron J. Schneider and David J. Kennedy

INTRODUCTION

- Upper limb sensory studies are commonly performed for detection and localization of multiple nerve pathologies, including peripheral mononeuropathies (median, ulnar, and radial), entrapment neuropathies, plexopathies, and generalized peripheral polyneuropathies.
- Studies are typically performed antidromically.
- To correctly perform and interpret these studies, it is essential to have a thorough understanding of both dermatomal and peripheral nerve distributions (Figure 5.1). Advanced studies, such as those used in the combined sensory index (CSI) and sensory studies (Table 5.1) in the forearm, are covered later.

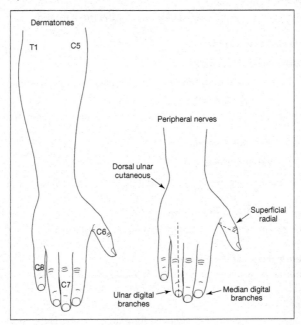

FIGURE 5.1 The innervation of the hand via dermatome map and peripheral nerve map.

Clinical Pearl
- Most radiculopathies occur due to pathology proximal to the dorsal root ganglion, resulting in normal sensory studies even when cervical radiculopathy is present.

MEDIAN TO INDEX OR MIDDLE FINGER
- May be abnormal due to medial or lateral cord pathology (Table 5.2), or median nerve compression commonly occurring at the carpal tunnel or less commonly at the pronator teres.
- The following are things to consider in the workup of carpal tunnel syndrome (CTS):
  - Is one of the digits more symptomatic? If so, use that digit for the study.
  - The most sensitive test for detecting CTS is the CSI.

TABLE 5.1 Sensory Branches: Median and Ulnar

Sensory Branches of the Ulnar Nerve
Palmar Ulnar Cutaneous (Before Guyon Canal)
• Supplies sensation to the medial aspect of the palm
Dorsal Ulnar Cutaneous (Before Guyon Canal)
• Supplies sensation to the medial aspect of the medial dorsum of the hand and the posterior aspect of the medial 1½ digits
Digital Branches (After Guyon Canal)
• Supplies sensation to the dorsal aspect and tips of the medial 1½ digits
Sensory Branches of the Median Nerve
Palmar Branch (Before Carpal Tunnel)
• Supplies sensation to the palm of the hand not affected in carpal tunnel syndrome
Digital Branches (After Carpal Tunnel)
• Supplies sensation to the palmar aspect and tips of the lateral 3½ fingers
Sensory Branches of the Radial Nerve
Posterior Cutaneous Nerve of the Arm
• Arises from the radial nerve in the axilla and innervates a small area on the lateral aspect of the shoulder
Lower Lateral Cutaneous Nerve of the Arm
• Arises from the radial nerve in the upper arm above the spiral groove and supplies the lateral arm
Posterior Cutaneous Nerve of the Forearm
• Arises from the radial nerve in the upper arm above the spiral groove and supplies the lateral arm
Superficial Radial Nerve
• Arises in the proximal forearm and supplies the skin of the dorsum of the hand and the lateral 3½ fingers

TABLE 5.2 Upper Limb Sensory

Test
Median to index or middle finger

Lead Placement

- E1: Ring electrode on the proximal phalanx
- E2: 3–4 cm distal to E1

Stimulation

- Wrist: 14 cm proximal to E1 between the tendons of the FCR and palmaris longus
- Midpalm: 7 cm proximal to E1 along the course of the median nerve

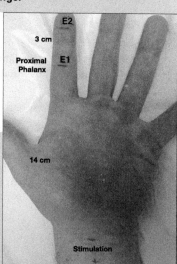

Test
Ulnar to little finger

Lead Placement

- E1: Ring electrode on the proximal phalanx
- E2: 3–4 cm distal to E1

Stimulation

- Wrist: 14 cm proximal to E1 on the medial aspect of the wrist adjacent to the flexor carpi ulnaris tendon

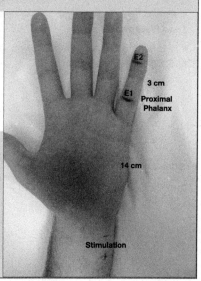

(*continued*)

TABLE 5.2 Upper Limb Sensory (*continued*)

Test
Dorsal ulnar cutaneous

Lead Placement

- Dorsal hand
- E1: Web space between the little and ring finger
- E2: 3–4 cm distal to E1 over the little finger

Stimulation

- Slightly proximal and inferior to the ulnar styloid with the hand pronated 10 cm proximal to E1

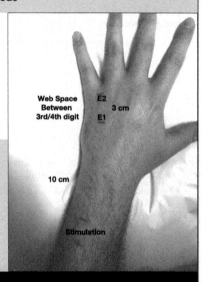

Test
Superficial radial

Lead Placement

- E1: Bar electrode on the first web space
- E2: 3–4 cm distal to E1

Stimulation

- Over the distal midradius 10 cm proximal to E1ww

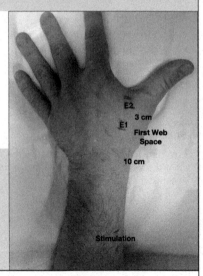

FCR, flexor carpi radialis.

ULNAR TO LITTLE FINGER
- May be abnormal due to lower trunk or medial cord pathology, or ulnar neuropathy (see Table 5.2).
- Stimulations above and below the elbow can be performed in the workup for ulnar neuropathy at the elbow. The sensory nerve study is more sensitive than the motor nerve study for detecting focal slowing across the elbow. However, due to temporal dispersion and phase cancellation, the amplitudes are not meaningful.

Clinical Pearls
- A volume-conducted motor potential may obscure the ulnar sensory potential.
- *Tip:* Ways to decrease conducted motor potential include placing the E1 ring electrode more distal on the finger and having the patient intentionally extend and abduct the 5th digit.

DORSAL ULNAR CUTANEOUS
- The dorsal ulnar cutaneous (DUC) nerve is useful in differentiating lesions at Guyon canal at the wrist from more proximal ulnar lesions (see Table 5.2).

SUPERFICIAL RADIAL
- May be abnormal due to upper or middle trunks and posterior cord pathology and in radial neuropathy (see Table 5.2).
- The superficial radial nerve can be palpated over the extensor pollicis longus tendon when the thumb is extended.

Clinical Pearl
- Using a ring electrode over the thumb allows for comparison to the median nerve to the thumb, which is used in the combined sensory index (CSI).

NORMAL VALUE RANGE
- There are a variety of normative values in the literature due to technique differences, patient population, and variations based on size and age; therefore, a range is presented here. Every laboratory should endeavor to have its own normal values based on the patient population. Initially, a textbook of normal values may be used.
  - Median nerve stimulating at the wrist and recording at digit 2 or 3
    - *Peak latency:* 3.5 to 3.6 ms
    - *Amplitude:* 6 to 10 μV
  - Ulnar nerve stimulating at the wrist and recording at digit 5
    - *Peak latency:* 3.6 to 3.8 ms
    - *Amplitude:* 6 to 17 μV

- Radial nerve stimulating at the wrist and recording at snuffbox
  - ☐ *Peak latency:* 2.9 to 3.1 ms
  - ☐ *Amplitude:* 7 to 15 μV

QUESTIONS

1. Decreased limb temperature has the following effects on sensory nerve action potentials:
   A. Decreased amplitude, increased (delayed) latency
   B. Decreased amplitude, decreased latency
   C. Increased amplitude, increased (delayed) latency
   D. Increased amplitude, decreased latency

2. Median nerve sensory study will be normal in:
   A. Carpal tunnel syndrome
   B. Medial cord brachial plexopathy
   C. Pronator teres entrapment neuropathy
   D. Cervical radiculopathy

3. Which of the following sensory studies is an example of orthodromic conduction?
   A. Median nerve with stimulation between the tendons of the flexor carpus radialis and palmaris longus and recording with ring electrodes at the index finger
   B. Ulnar nerve with stimulation at medial aspect of the wrist adjacent to the flexor carpi ulnaris tendon and recording with ring electrodes at the little finger
   C. Radial nerve with stimulation at the distal radius and recording with bar electrode at the first web space
   D. Ulnar nerve transpalmar study with stimulation between the fourth and fifth metacarpals and recording on the medial aspect of the wrist adjacent to the flexor carpi ulnaris tendon

4. Peak latency of median nerve study is 4.0 ms. Potential causes for this include all of the following EXCEPT:
   A. Limb temperature is too cold
   B. Stimulation occurred at 18 cm
   C. Patient has carpal tunnel syndrome
   D. Patient has amyotrophic lateral sclerosis

5. The dorsal ulnar cutaneous nerve is useful in differentiating:
   A. Tarsal tunnel syndrome from carpal tunnel syndrome
   B. Lesions at Guyon canal at the wrist from more proximal ulnar lesions
   C. Pronator teres syndrome from C7 radiculopathy
   D. Ulnar neuropathy at the elbow from lateral cord brachial plexopathy

---

Answers to the questions are located in Chapter 35.

ADDITIONAL READINGS

American Association of Electrodiagnostic Medicine, American Academy of Neurology, American Academy of Physical Medicine and Rehabilitation. Practice parameter for electrodiagnostic studies in ulnar neuropathy at the elbow: summary statement. *Muscle Nerve.* 1999;22(3):408–411. PubMed PMID: 10086904.

Buschbacher RM. Median 14-cm and 7-cm antidromic sensory studies to digits two and three. *Am J Phys Med Rehabil.* 1999;78(6 suppl):S53–S62. PubMed PMID: 10573099.

Buschbacher RM. Ulnar 14-cm and 7-cm antidromic sensory studies to the fifth digit: reference values derived from a large population of normal subjects. *Am J Phys Med Rehabil.* 1999;78(6 suppl):S63–S68. PubMed PMID: 10573100.

Lew HL, Tsai SJ. Pictorial guide to muscles and surface anatomy. In: Pease WS, Lew HL, Johnson EW, eds. *Johnson's Practical Electromyography.* 4th ed. Philadelphia, PA: Lippincott Williams & Wilkins; 2007:231–238.

Mackenzie K, DeLisa JA. Distal sensory latency measurement of the superficial radial nerve in normal adult subjects. *Arch Phys Med Rehabil.* 1981;62(1):31–34. PubMed PMID: 7458630.

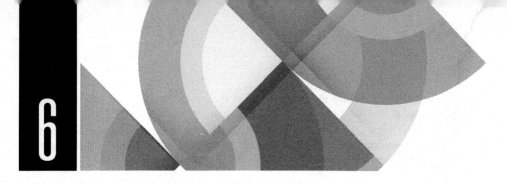

Lower Limb Motor Studies

Berdale Colorado

INTRODUCTION

- Tibial and fibular (peroneal) motor nerve conduction studies (NCSs) are used in most lower limb electrodiagnostic evaluations and should be mastered early.
- Begin by reviewing anatomy to facilitate understanding that:
  - The sciatic nerve is formed by the ventral rami of L4 through S3.
  - In the popliteal fossa, it divides into the tibial and common fibular nerves.
  - The tibial nerve innervates the muscles of the posterior leg and then divides posterior and distal to the medial malleolus into the medial and lateral plantar nerves innervating the sole of the foot.
  - The common fibular nerve leaves the popliteal fossa and courses toward the fibular head/neck. This is a common site of injury and the general area of the separation into the deep and superficial fibular nerves, which innervate the muscles of the anterior and lateral leg, respectively.

FIBULAR (PERONEAL) TO EXTENSOR DIGITORUM BREVIS

- The deep fibular nerve innervates the extensor digitorum brevis (EDB) (Table 6.1).
- The motor study may be abnormal with any injury of the sciatic, common fibular, or deep fibular nerve.
- A deep fibular motor study to the tibialis anterior may be employed when the EDB is atrophied, as may occur in a peripheral neuropathy or in an L5–S1 radiculopathy with axonal loss.

Troubleshooting

- Avoid co-stimulation of the tibial nerve at the popliteal fossa (look for ankle plantarflexion).
- The majority of isolated injuries to this nerve occur at the fibular head/neck; ensure adequate distance between the below-fibular head and popliteal fossa stimulation sites for more accurate determination of the conduction velocity.

- Higher stimulation intensity may be needed at the below-fibular head site because the nerve is deeper at that location.
- A higher compound muscle action potential (CMAP) amplitude at the below-fibular head and popliteal fossa stimulation sites compared to the ankle stimulation site should raise suspicion for the presence of an accessory fibular (peroneal) nerve.

TABLE 6.1 Fibular (Peroneal) Motor to Extensor Digitorum Brevis

Lead Placement
• E1: Midpoint of the extensor digitorum brevis on the dorsum of the foot • E2: At the distal myotendinous junction (pictured) or at the 5th metatarsophalangeal joint • G: Dorsum of the foot
Stimulation
• S1—Ankle: 8 cm proximal to the E1, lateral to the tibialis anterior tendon • S2—Below-fibular head: Posterior and inferior to the fibular head • S3—Above-fibular head: Lateral popliteal fossa, just medial to the biceps femoris tendon

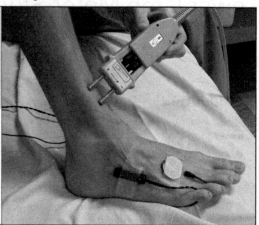

TIBIAL TO ABDUCTOR HALLUCIS

- The tibial nerve (medial plantar branch) innervates the abductor hallucis (AH) (Table 6.2).
- The motor study may be abnormal with any injury of the sciatic, tibial, or medial plantar nerve.

TABLE 6.2 Tibial Motor to Abductor Hallucis

Lead Placement
• E1: Medial foot, just anterior and inferior to the navicular tubercle • E2: At the 1st metatarsophalangeal joint • G: Dorsum of the foot
Stimulation
• S1—8 cm proximal to E1, just posterior to the medial malleolus • S2—Midpopliteal fossa

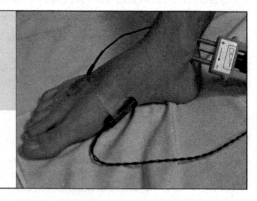

Troubleshooting
- Isolated injury to the tibial nerve is rare.
- Avoid co-stimulation of the fibular nerve at the popliteal fossa (look for ankle dorsiflexion and eversion).
- Higher stimulation intensity may be needed at the popliteal fossa because the nerve is deeper at that location.
- CMAP amplitude at the popliteal fossa stimulation site is typically lower than at the ankle stimulation site (up to 50% drop may still be normal); therefore, use caution when labeling as abnormal. Consider comparison to the other side.

REFERENCE VALUES
- The Normative Data Task Force of the American Association of Neuromuscular and Electrodiagnostic Medicine (2016) identified only one fibular motor nerve study and two tibial motor nerve studies in the literature that were considered suitable as a resource for NCS metrics (1). The recommended reference values are:

Fibular Nerve
- Onset latency: 6.5 ms
- Amplitude: 1.3 mV

Tibial Nerve
- Onset latency: 6.1 ms
- Amplitude: 4.4 mV

QUESTIONS

1. Despite a proper setup, stimulating at the popliteal fossa and below-fibular head sites for the fibular motor study to the extensor digitorum brevis reveals CMAP amplitudes higher than the CMAP amplitude when stimulating at the ankle. To evaluate for an accessory fibular nerve, you would stimulate:
   A. Midline posterior calf, about 14 cm from the ankle
   B. Anterolateral lower leg, about 14 cm from the ankle
   C. Posterior to the lateral malleolus
   D. Posterior to the medial malleolus

2. While preparing for an electrodiagnostic examination, you palpate a popliteal cyst in the popliteal fossa. Which nerve would most likely be affected by this finding?
   A. Sciatic
   B. Common fibular
   C. Sural sensory
   D. Tibial

Answers to the questions are located in Chapter 35.

3. While performing a routine tibial motor study to the abductor hallucis, you notice an initial positive deflection of the CMAP waveform. The most likely cause of this deflection is:
   A. The E1 electrode is not over the motor endplate
   B. Accessory tibial nerve is present
   C. Insufficient stimulation intensity in the popliteal fossa
   D. Co-stimulation of the fibular nerve

4. While performing a routine tibial motor study to the abductor hallucis, you notice a CMAP amplitude drop of 40% at the popliteal fossa stimulation site compared to the ankle stimulation site. This finding is most likely:
   A. A conduction block
   B. Co-stimulation of the fibular nerve
   C. Evidence of an accessory tibial nerve
   D. Within normal limits

REFERENCE

1. Chen S, Andary M, Buschbacher R, et al. Electrodiagnostic reference values for upper and lower limb nerve conduction studies in adult populations. *Muscle Nerve*. 2016;54:371–377. doi:10.1002/mus.25203

Lower Limb Sensory Studies

Jacqueline Neal and Nida Gleveckas-Martens

INTRODUCTION
- General considerations for performing nerve conduction studies:
  - Prepare skin: No lotion should be used; mildly abrade skin with an alcohol pad.
  - Attention must be paid to technical issues, such as skin temperature, measurements, and setup, as variations from the setup for published normative data may invalidate the reference values.
    - As a general standard, a temperature greater than 32°C recorded on the dorsum of the foot is recommended.
    - Recommend use of a low-frequency filter at 20 Hz and a high-frequency filter at 2 kHz.
  - Always be mindful of potential anatomic variations.
  - Given the nature of sensory responses, focus closely on obtaining supramaximal stimulation while ensuring avoidance of stimulus artifacts and co-stimulation of nearby nerves.
    - Sensory nerve action potential (SNAP) should be reproducible in amplitude and latency across multiple stimuli.
    - Width of negative phase is typically less than 2 ms; if duration is longer, the response may be artifactual.
    - If the SNAP onset latency is difficult to determine because of baseline artifact, average 10 to 20 responses.
  - Eliciting a SNAP may be challenging in patients with pedal edema, excess fatty tissue, or in those who are older in age.
  - Most studies are performed antidromically.
  - A SNAP is biphasic or triphasic. Both onset latency and peak latency can be measured/compared. Side-to-side comparison is helpful.
- Lower extremity nerve conduction studies are useful for evaluating for neuropathic lesions involving and distal to the dorsal root ganglion.
  - Typically, lesions proximal to the dorsal root ganglion (i.e., radiculopathies) lead to normal SNAPs.
  - Keeping in mind lower extremity dermatomes and peripheral cutaneous innervation is useful to help with localizing a lesion. See Figure 7.1 for a dermatomal map.

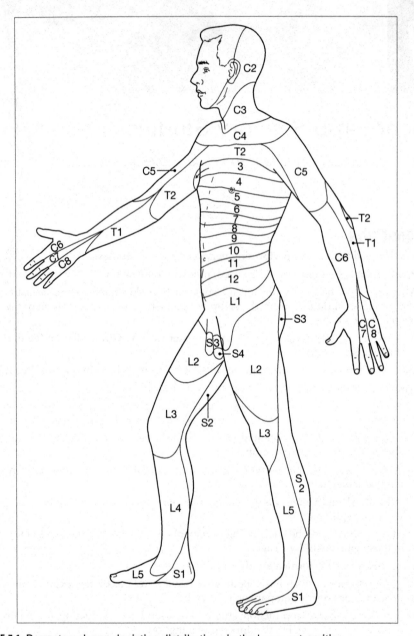

FIGURE 7.1 Dermatomal map depicting distributions in the lower extremities.

Source: Adapted from Haymaker W, Woodhall B. *Peripheral Nerve Injuries*. Philadelphia, PA: WB Saunders Company; 1945:20, Figure 15.

SCIATIC NERVE

- **Anatomy** (Figure 7.2)
  - Leaves the spine at L4–S3 roots
  - Forms a single trunk, though divisible into tibial and common peroneal components
  - Exits the pelvis through the greater sciatic foramen, emerging in the gluteal region
  - Travels laterally and downward midway between the ischial tuberosity and the greater trochanter deep to the gluteus maximus
  - Descends the thigh between the adductor magnus and hamstring muscles, and terminates just above the popliteal fossa by dividing into the tibial and common peroneal nerves

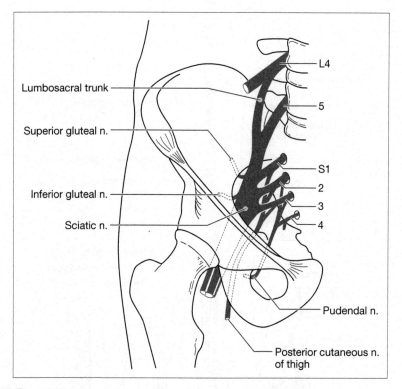

FIGURE 7.2 The sciatic nerve pathway in the pelvis and upper thigh.

Source: Adapted from Haymaker W, Woodhall B. *Peripheral Nerve Injuries.* Philadelphia, PA: WB Saunders Company; 1945:193, Figure 201.

SURAL NERVE

- **Anatomy** (Figure 7.3)
  - Most often made up of two components: Medial component from the tibial nerve and lateral component from the common peroneal nerve

44 | Nerve Conduction Studies

- In up to 25% of subjects, the sural nerve may be made up of components from the tibial or common peroneal nerves alone
- Sural nerve emerges from the gastrocnemius muscle near the musculotendinous junction of the gastrocnemius, then penetrates a fibrous arcade, which is a point that may rarely be compressed

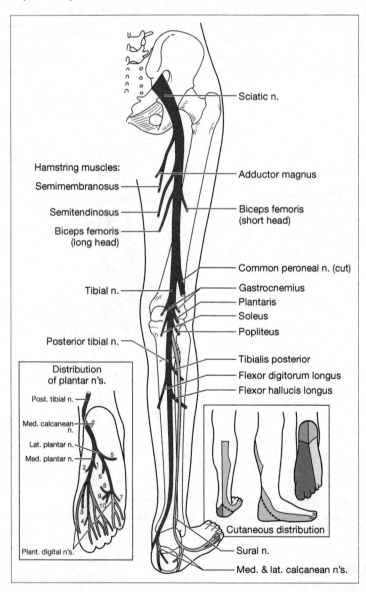

FIGURE 7.3 The sural nerve pathway as well as cutaneous distribution.

Source: Adapted from Haymaker W, Woodhall B. *Peripheral Nerve Injuries.* Philadelphia, PA: WB Saunders Company; 1945:196, Figure 203.

- **Setup** (Figure 7.4)
    - Instrumentation settings:
        - Sensitivity 2 to 5 µV per division; sweep 1 ms/div
    - Recording electrode: Use a bar electrode; place posterior inferior to the lateral malleolus (G1 electrode proximal, G2 electrode distal)
    - Place ground between stimulation and recording electrodes
    - Stimulate 14 cm proximal to G1 in the midline of the calf, or slightly lateral to midline

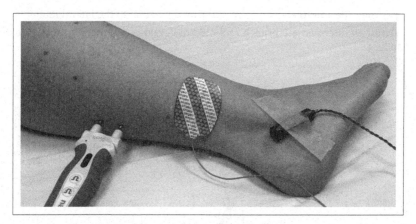

FIGURE 7.4 Sural nerve conduction setup.

- **Normative data (1)**
    - Onset-to-peak and peak-to-peak amplitude: Greater than 4 µV
    - Peak latency: Less than 4.5 ms; onset latency: less than 3.6 ms
    - Conduction velocity: Greater than 40 m/sec
    - Side-to-side latency difference of more than 0.5 ms is significant
    - Side-to-side amplitude difference of 40% or more is likely significant
- **Pearls**
    - Most normal older adults (98%) should have a sural response and absence of a response is likely pathological
    - Amplitudes decline with age
    - Latencies and velocities are mildly slower as age increases, but in a statistically insignificant fashion
    - May be abnormal in lumbosacral plexopathies, sciatic mononeuropathies, injuries to the tibial nerve, and polyneuropathies.
        - Should be normal in radiculopathies
        - Direct compressive neuropathy of the sural nerve is rare

SUPERFICIAL FIBULAR (PERONEAL) NERVE

- **Anatomy** (Figure 7.5)
  - Leaves the spine at L5 nerve root and travels through the lumbosacral plexus
  - Down the posterior thigh in the sciatic nerve-peroneal division
  - Across the knee as the common fibular (peroneal) nerve
  - Branches to the superficial fibular (peroneal) nerve after crossing the fibular head
  - Travels down the lateral leg between the peroneus longus and brevis, piercing the deep fascia and becoming superficial at the lower third of the leg
  - Crosses over the anterolateral aspect of the ankle medial to the lateral malleolus
  - Splits into an intermediate branch and medial dorsal cutaneous branch in the dorsum of the foot

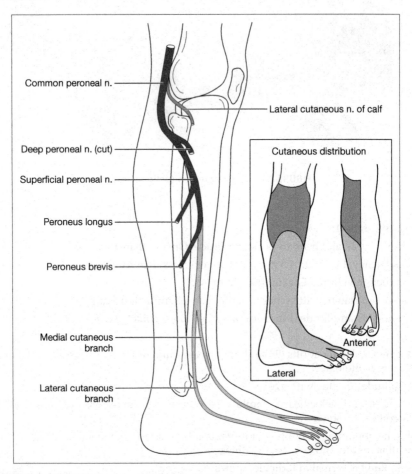

FIGURE 7.5 Superficial fibular (peroneal) nerve pathway as well as cutaneous distribution.

Source: Adapted from Haymaker W, Woodhall B. *Peripheral Nerve Injuries*. Philadelphia, PA: WB Saunders Company; 1945:198, Figure 204.

- **Setup** (Figure 7.6)
  - Instrumentation settings
    - Gain 20 µV/div and sweep 2 ms/div
  - Recommend using the Izzo technique (2,3)
    - Recording electrode: Utilize a bar electrode; place over the medial dorsal cutaneous nerve at the level of the anterior ankle with G1 electrode proximal and G2 electrode distal
      - Palpation of the superficial fibular (peroneal) nerve at the anterior ankle with the ankle placed in plantarflexion and inversion can help with localizing placement for G1 electrode
    - Place ground between stimulation and recording electrodes
    - Stimulate 14 cm proximal to G1 over the course of the superficial fibular (peroneal) nerve at the anterolateral leg
      - To localize the superficial fibular (peroneal) nerve at the anterolateral leg, direct a measuring tape from G1 up to the fibular head, and the path of the measuring tape will roughly demonstrate the path of the superficial peroneal nerve

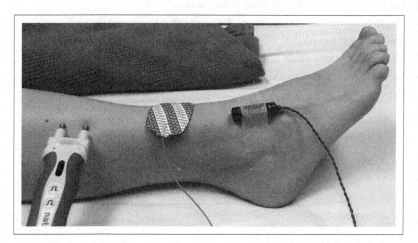

FIGURE 7.6 Superficial fibular (peroneal) nerve conduction study setup.

- **Normative data (2)**
  - High-quality normative data are not available
  - Suggest using the following reference values with strong recommendation for side-to-side comparison
    - Onset-to-peak amplitude: 3.8 µV
    - Peak latency: Less than 3.4 ms
    - Conduction velocity: Greater than 40.7 m/s

- **Pearls**
  - Common compression sites include the fibular head and much less often the ankle.
  - Can record over the medial or intermediate branches; most commonly recorded at the intermediate branch.
  - Up to 11% of the population will demonstrate no response.
  - Medial dorsal cutaneous branch has more data available.
  - May be abnormal in lesions of the lumbosacral plexus, sciatic nerve, common peroneal nerve, isolated superficial peroneal compressive neuropathies, peripheral neuropathies, and occasionally in L5 radiculopathies.

SAPHENOUS

- **Anatomy** (Figure 7.7)
  - Leaves the spine at the L4 nerve root
  - Travels through the lumbosacral plexus
  - Down the anterior thigh, traveling with the femoral artery
  - Diverges from the femoral artery as it passes the adductor magnus
  - Descends along the medial side of the knee behind the sartorius
  - Passes along the tibial side of the leg behind the medial border of the tibia
  - Cutaneous innervation to the medial leg, ankle, and foot

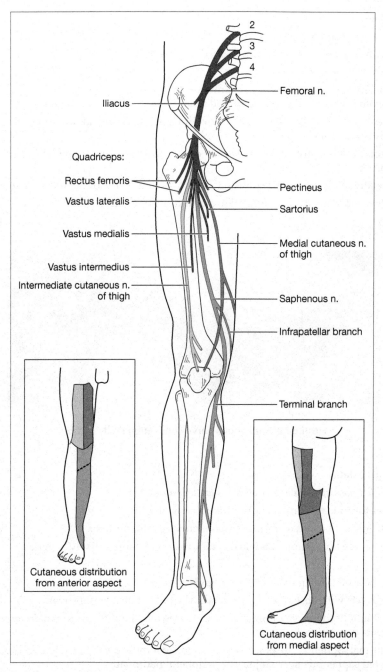

FIGURE 7.7 Saphenous nerve pathway and cutaneous distribution.

Source: Adapted from Haymaker W, Woodhall B. *Peripheral Nerve Injuries*. Philadelphia, PA: WB Saunders Company; 1945:189, Figure 197.

- **Setup** (Figure 7.8)
  - Instrumentation settings:
    - Gain 2 to 5 µV/div and sweep speed of 1 ms/div
  - Patient lying supine
  - 3-cm bar electrode placed just anterior to the highest prominence of the medial malleolus, between the malleolus and tibialis anterior tendon
    - Reference electrode (G2) at the level of the malleolus, and active electrode (G1) proximal to that
  - Stimulate 14 cm proximal to the active electrode just medial to the most medial aspect of the tibia
    - Relatively deep pressure directed toward the underside of the tibia is suggested
  - Ground placed between stimulation site and active electrode

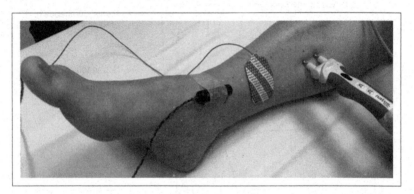

FIGURE 7.8 Saphenous nerve conduction study setup.

- **Normative data**
  - *Note that normative data were obtained without averaging*
  - Onset-to-peak amplitude: 2 µV; peak-to-peak amplitude: 1 µV
  - Peak latency: Less than 4.4 ms; onset latency: less than 3.8 ms
  - Side-to-side amplitude difference of 65% to 78% or more is likely significant
- **Pearls**
  - May be absent in up to 25% of the population.
    - Subjects with absent responses tend to be older, taller, and heavier.
  - Small amplitudes are common and responses may be difficult to obtain, especially in patients older than 40.
  - Abnormal saphenous responses can be found in lumbar plexopathy, femoral neuropathy, isolated saphenous nerve injury, or peripheral neuropathy.

LATERAL FEMORAL CUTANEOUS NERVE

- **Anatomy** (Figure 7.9)
  - Pure sensory nerve
  - Formed from ventral divisions of L2/3 nerve roots
  - Travels deep intra-abdominally, over the lateral border of the psoas, medial to anterior superior iliac spine (ASIS), under or through the inguinal ligament
  - Usually innervates the lateral portion of the thigh, but in some may also innervate parts of the anterior thigh (variable anatomy)

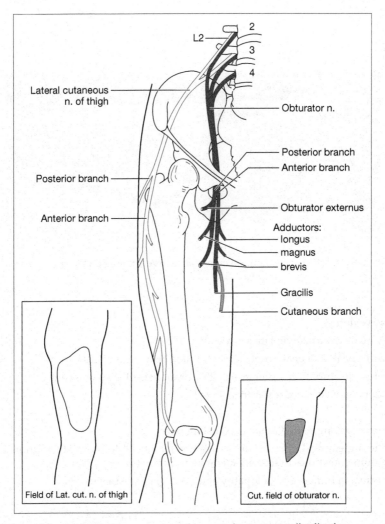

FIGURE 7.9 Lateral femoral cutaneous nerve pathway and cutaneous distribution.

Source: Adapted from Haymaker W, Woodhall B. *Peripheral Nerve Injuries*. Philadelphia, PA: WB Saunders Company; 1945:186, Figure 195.

- **Setup** (Figure 7.10)
    - ☐ Instrumentation setting recommendations are not described in the literature; authors recommend the following: Gain 2 to 5 µV/div and sweep speed of 1 ms/div
- Recording electrode: Use a bar electrode; place G1 electrode proximal, G2 electrode distal
    - ☐ G1 placed 12 cm distal to the ASIS along a line from the ASIS to the lateral border of the patella; may need to move bar electrode medial to this point if no response is recordable
- Place ground between stimulation and recording electrodes
- Stimulate 1 to 1.5 cm distal and medial to the ASIS

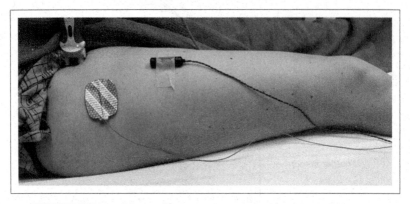

FIGURE 7.10 Lateral femoral cutaneous nerve conduction study setup.

- **Normative data**
    - High-quality normative data are not available
    - Onset-to-peak and peak-to-peak amplitude: Greater than 3 µV
    - Side-to-side amplitude difference of 45% or more is likely significant
    - Conduction velocity: Greater than 45 m/s
- **Pearls**
    - Commonly compressed at the inguinal ligament
    - Due to a great deal of anatomic variability, may need to move stimulation/recording sites numerous times to find an adequate response (4)
    - Abnormal in lumbar radiculopathy and meralgia paresthetica

QUESTIONS

1. Reduced amplitudes in both the superficial peroneal sensory nerve and the sural sensory nerve would help with localizing a lesion where?
   A. Common peroneal nerve
   B. Sciatic nerve
   C. Femoral nerve
   D. Lumbar plexus

2. In a patient with abnormal femoral motor nerve conduction studies and absent responses in saphenous nerve conduction studies, which would be the most likely lesion localization?
   A. Saphenous nerve
   B. Lumbar radiculopathy
   C. Femoral nerve
   D. None of the above

3. The lateral femoral cutaneous nerve response may be absent in:
   A. Meralgia paresthetica, L5 radiculopathy
   B. Meralgia paresthetica, L3 radiculopathy
   C. Meralgia paresthetica, femoral mononeuropathy
   D. Meralgia paresthetica, lumbar plexopathy

4. Which lower extremity sensory response may be abnormal in a patient with a lumbosacral radiculopathy?
   A. Lateral femoral cutaneous
   B. Saphenous
   C. Superficial peroneal
   D. Sural

5. The sural nerve:
   A. Contains fibers originating in the L4 root
   B. Is composed of axons originating in the common peroneal and tibial nerves
   C. Innervates the entire plantar aspect of the foot
   D. Supplies the peroneus longus muscle

6. A patient complains of anterior thigh pain and weakness, as well as numbness/paresthesia on the anterior thigh and medial leg. Which lower extremity sensory nerve conduction study would be most useful to perform?
   A. Sural
   B. Saphenous
   C. Superficial peroneal
   D. Lateral femoral cutaneous

Answers to the questions are located in Chapter 35.

ADDITIONAL READINGS

Chen S, Andary M, Buschbacher R, et al. Electrodiagnostic reference values for upper and lower limb nerve conduction studies in adult populations. *Muscle Nerve*. 2016;54:371–377. doi:10.1002/mus.25203

Dillingham T, Chen S, Andary M, et al. Establishing high quality reference values for nerve conduction studies: a report from the normative data task force of the American Association of Neuromuscular and Electrodiagnostic Medicine. *Muscle Nerve*. 2016;54:366–370. doi:10.1002/mus.25204

REFERENCES

1. Buschbacher RM. Sural and saphenous 14-cm antidromic sensory nerve conduction studies. *Am J Phys Med Rehabil*. 2003;82:421–426. PubMed PMID: 12820783.
2. Falco FJ, Hennessey WJ, Goldberg G, et al. Standardized nerve conduction studies in the lower limb of the healthy elderly. *Am J Phys Med Rehabil*. 1994;73:168–174. PubMed PMID: 8198773.
3. Izzo KL, Sridhara CR, Rosenholtz H, et al. Sensory conduction studies of the branches of the superficial peroneal nerve. *Arch Phys Med Rehabil*. 1981;62(1):24–27. PubMed PMID: 7458628.
4. Shin YB, Park JH, Kwon DR, et al. Variability in conduction of the lateral femoral cutaneous nerve. *Muscle Nerve*. 2006;33:645–649. doi:10.1002/mus.20505.

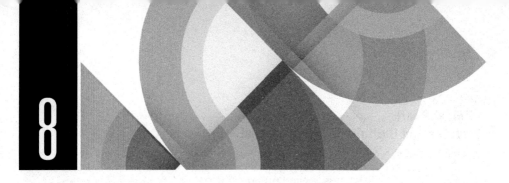

8

F-Waves

Solomon Rojhani and Akhil Chhatre

INTRODUCTION

- F-waves and H-reflexes are known as *late responses*. Late responses evaluate the **entire nerve** from root to the neuromuscular junction.
- Routine nerve conduction studies (NCSs) only test the distal segment of peripheral nerves. F-waves represent the antidromic motor responses obtained following electrical stimulation of a peripheral nerve.
- They are most useful when the distal segment is normal and the proximal segment is abnormal. Measuring a longer segment allows detection of a proximal or diffuse problem, such as a demyelinating process.
  - Assessing a nerve using the distal segment is comparable to trying to assess the performance of a marathoner by only observing the final mile of his or her run and assuming that the final mile accurately represents what happened for the prior 25 miles.
  - Although this may be true for many runners, there are some instances when you want to see what happened for the first 25 miles.
  - Similarly, with many nerve studies (e.g., assessing for carpal tunnel syndrome), we are primarily interested in the distal nerve segments.
  - However, there are several specific examples for which it would be valuable to measure the time required traversing the proximal nerve segment. F-waves are used to measure the entire nerve segment and reflect that time.
    - ☐ Early acute inflammatory demyelinating polyneuropathy/Guillain–Barré syndrome (selectively demyelinates proximally)
    - ☐ Possibly in C8–T1 and L5–S1 radiculopathies
    - ☐ Lumbar spinal stenosis after walking—increased chronodispersion
    - ☐ Early peripheral polyneuropathy when more distal NCS are normal
    - ☐ Entrapment neuropathies (control values)
    - ☐ Increased billing/revenue potential is *not* an acceptable reason to perform F-waves

Clinical Pearl
F-Waves and Guillain–Barré Syndrome
- One condition for which F-waves are useful is Guillain–Barré syndrome (GBS). GBS is a segmental demyelinating disorder that results in ascending weakness starting with the distal muscles and progressing to the more proximal muscles. Early in the course of GBS, the nerve roots are often preferentially affected. Therefore, in early GBS the only abnormality may be delayed F-waves. This makes them a crucial part of the diagnosis.

ANATOMY
- The F-response is not an actual reflex; a reflex is a response that goes through a sensory component, synapses in the central nervous system, and then travels back down into the motor pathway. With F-waves, the pathway is from motor fiber to cell body and back to motor fiber.
- The impulse first propagates proximally (antidromically) along the motor nerve to the cell body in the anterior horn.
  - As the impulse approaches the cell body, the membrane at the most proximal part of the axon where it meets the cell body (axon hillock) is the first part of the cell body to see the impulse and the first part to recover after the refractory period. Blocking of this antidromic potential usually occurs at the hillock.
  - The signal travels around the rest of the cell and essentially circles back to the axon hillock.
  - The timing is such that a very small percentage of motor neurons get reactivated and send an impulse back down the motor pathway orthodromically—about 1% to 2%.
- To get this 1% to 2% bounce back, you need to stimulate **all** of the motor fibers, requiring supramaximal stimulation (this is in contrast to the H-reflex, which requires submaximal stimulation, Table 8.1).
  - The response you get is actually very small—about 1% to 5% of the compound muscle action potential.
  - Because it was detected first in the foot, this response is given the name "F"-wave.
    - ☐ Recommended reading: Dumitru's textbook discusses the interesting physiology of the F-wave in much more detail (1).

TABLE 8.1 Comparison of F-Waves and H-Reflexes

	F-Waves	H-Reflexes
Pathway	Antidromic (motor afferent) and orthodromic (motor efferent)	Orthodromic (sensory afferent) and orthodromic (motor efferent)
Stimulation	Supramaximal	Submaximal with increased duration pulse
Amplitude	50–300 µV	10–30 µV
Latency	28–34 ms median/ulnar and 50–56 ms peroneal/tibial (variable; age and height/limb-length dependent)	28–36 ms (variable; age and height/limb-length dependent)
Miscellaneous	Compare symptomatic side to asymptomatic side	Compare side-to-side values; 1.5–2.0 ms difference is acceptable

ELECTRODIAGNOSTIC APPROACH

- The setup for an F-wave is very similar to that of a routine motor NCS.
  - Flip the stimulator so the cathode (black) is proximal and the anode (gray) is distal. This is to prevent theoretical anodal block (Figure 8.1).
  - Stimulation intensity is gradually increased until supramaximal stimulation intensity is obtained. Then, a series of waveforms are recorded on a rastered trace, usually at least 8 to 10 (Figure 8.2). Modern electrodiagnostic software allows for averaging of F-wave traces.
  - Each of the F responses obtained represents different fibers and, therefore, will vary somewhat in latency, configuration, and amplitude (see Figure 8.2).
  - After performing all of the F-waves, look for a normal pattern:
    - **Mark the minimal F-wave latency:** This is most commonly used. Presumably, the fastest recording represents the largest and fastest motor fibers. Check against normative values—taller individuals will have longer latencies.
    - **Count the persistence:** This is defined as the number of F-waves obtained divided by the number of stimulations. Use of persistence is controversial. Fibular (peroneal) F-waves normally have low persistence.
    - **Measure the chronodispersion:** This is defined as the difference between the fastest and the slowest F-waves obtained. There is some evidence of increased chronodispersion in lumbar spinal stenosis after subjects walk or stand for 3 minutes and become symptomatic (2).
    - **F-wave mean latency:** The mean of at least seven F-wave latencies (3). This reflects the average of the recorded F-waves. Potentially the most accurate measurement for clinical applications.

58 | Nerve Conduction Studies

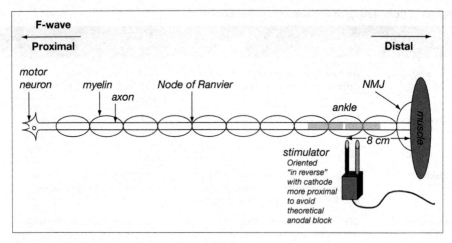

FIGURE 8.1

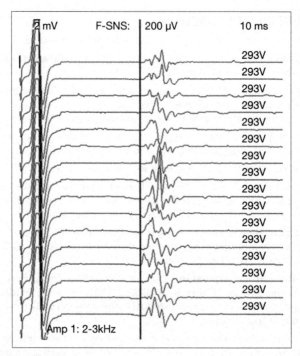

FIGURE 8.2 Measure the chronodispersion: This is the difference between the fastest and the slowest F-waves obtained.

LIMITATIONS

- F-waves test the entire length of the peripheral nerve. An abnormal F-wave does not indicate where along the pathway the pathology lies.
- F-waves test only the nerve roots that innervate the muscles tested. In the upper limb, F-waves are most often performed with the median and ulnar nerves, which are innervated by C8 and T1. In the lower limb, they are usually performed with the fibular (peroneal) and tibial nerves, which are L5–S1.
- F-waves test only motor nerve fibers.
- Peroneal F-waves may be absent in normals.
- F-waves may be absent in sleeping or sedated patients, and in cases where distal motor unit amplitude is reduced.
- For the F-wave to be absent or for the minimal latency to be delayed, all or most of the fibers have to be affected.

QUESTIONS

1. How large is the F-wave compared to the compound muscle action potentials for the muscle being studied?
   A. Less than 1%
   B. 1% to 5%
   C. 5% to 10%
   D. 10% to 15%

2. Which of the presenting complaints could be an indication for using F-waves?
   A. Flick sign
   B. Ascending weakness
   C. Pain at the great toe
   D. Numbness of the first web space of the hand

3. Which describes the afferent limb of the F-wave?
   A. Antidromic motor
   B. Antidromic sensory
   C. Orthodromic motor
   D. Orthodromic sensory

4. Which represents the largest and fastest motor fibers?
   A. Persistence
   B. Chronodispersion
   C. Anodal block
   D. Minimal F-wave latency

Answers to the questions are located in Chapter 35.

5. In which clinical condition would F-waves be of least clinical value?
   A. Peripheral polyneuropathy
   B. Acute inflammatory demyelinating polyneuropathy
   C. L5–S1 radiculopathy
   D. Meralgia paresthetica (lateral femoral cutaneous neuropathy)

6. All of the following statements regarding F-waves are true except:
   A. F-waves are obtained by using a supramaximal stimulus
   B. The shortest F-wave latency represents the largest and fastest conducting fibers
   C. The F-wave initially begins with orthodromic stimulation of sensory fibers and represents a true reflex
   D. F-wave latency is directly related to height, limb length, and age

REFERENCES
1. Dumitru D. *Electrodiagnostic Medicine*. 2nd ed. Philadelphia, PA: Hanley & Belfus; 2002:238–241.
2. Tang LM, Schwartz MS, Swash M. Postural effects on F-wave parameters in lumbosacral root compression and canal stenosis. *Brain*. 1988;207:207–213. PubMed PMID: 2966648.
3. Medrati F, Vecchierini MF. F-waves: neurophysiology and clinical value. *Neurophysiol Clin*. 2004;34(5):217–243. doi:10.1016/j.neucli.2004.09.005

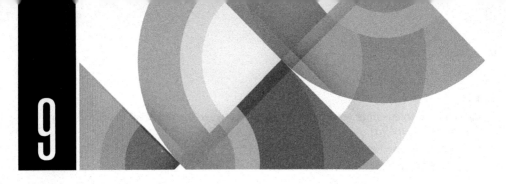

H-Reflexes

Leslie Rydberg

INTRODUCTION

The H-reflex is a monosynaptic reflex that was first described by Hoffman in 1918. It can be used for:

- S1 radiculopathy: This is the most common use of the H-reflex; it assesses the conduction properties of the S1 nerve root in the neural foramen to investigate the possibility of nerve root compromise, which would lead to an increased latency (slowing)
- Cervical radiculopathy/brachial plexopathy: The H-reflex can be tested in the flexor carpi radialis (FCR) to assess the C6 and C7 nerve roots
- Polyneuropathy
- Guillain–Barré syndrome
- Tibial or sciatic neuropathy, lumbosacral plexopathy

ANATOMY

- Orthodromic sensory afferent (Ia muscle spindle afferents), carrying the impulse to the spinal cord
- A synapse in the spinal cord (at the anterior horn cell or interneuron)
- Orthodromic motor efferent (alpha motor neuron) carrying the impulse to the muscle and completing the arc
- The H-reflex represents a delayed motor response

ELECTRODIAGNOSTIC APPROACH

Unlike the F-wave, which can be obtained with any peripheral motor nerve, the H-reflex is only routinely obtained at the soleus muscle. Here, the H-reflex travels along the tibial nerve and assesses only the S1 fibers. It is the electrical correlate of the gastroc–soleus muscle stretch reflex tested at the Achilles tendon. It can also be performed with the FCR, but this is not commonly done.

Setup
- E1: Over the soleus muscle measured halfway between the popliteal fossa and the medial malleolus (Figure 9.1)
- E2: Over the posterior calcaneus
- Ground: Proximal to the active electrode

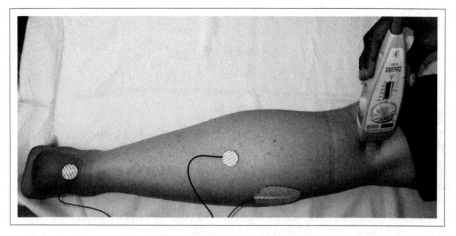

FIGURE 9.1 Setup for H-reflex.

- Stimulation: In the popliteal fossa with the anode distal to the cathode; both the sensory Ia afferent and the alpha motor neuron efferent in the tibial nerve are stimulated simultaneously
- Duration: 1 ms (long duration current)
- Stimulus intensity: Submaximal stimulus

Performing the Study
- Successive stimulations are performed while gradually increasing the intensity (Figure 9.2).
  - The goal is to find the stimulus intensity that will give the maximal H-reflex amplitude and minimal latency.
  - The cursor is then placed at the point that marks the minimal latency.
    - The minimal H latency is the most commonly used measure and is usually compared side to side or can be compared to the normal population.
    - The latency varies with leg length (or height) and age. The upper limit of normal latency ranges from 30.0 to 38.2 ms depending on age and height.
    - Normally, there is less than 1.2 ms difference from side to side.
- At low-stimulation intensities the Ia sensory afferents are preferentially stimulated and only an H-reflex will be seen.
- As the stimulation intensity gradually increases, the H-reflex amplitude increases and the latency decreases.

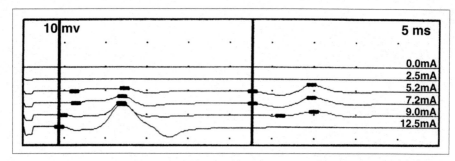

FIGURE 9.2

As the intensity is increased further, the M-wave begins to appear and the amplitude of the H-reflex decreases. At higher intensities, the H-reflex disappears and the M-wave predominates.

QUESTIONS

1. Which of the following represents the correct pathway of the H-reflex arc?
   A. Orthodromic sensory Ia afferents → Orthodromic alpha motor neuron efferents
   B. Antidromic sensory Ia afferents → Orthodromic alpha motor neuron efferents
   C. Antidromic alpha motor neuron afferents → Orthodromic alpha motor neuron efferents
   D. Orthodromic alpha motor neuron afferents → Orthodromic sensory Ia efferents

2. Which of the following statements regarding the H-reflex is **correct**?
   A. An H-reflex requires a supramaximal stimulus.
   B. The H-reflex amplitude is constant at all stimulus levels.
   C. The H-reflex is caused by a polysynaptic reflex.
   D. The latency difference compared between left and right legs in an H-reflex should be less than 2 ms.

3. A 70-year-old man has a significantly prolonged H-reflex on the right and a normal H-reflex on the left. What is the most likely diagnosis?
   A. Right sciatic neuropathy
   B. Guillain–Barré syndrome
   C. Polyneuropathy
   D. Right S1 radiculopathy

ADDITIONAL READING

Dumitru D. *Electrodiagnostic Medicine*. 2nd ed. Philadelphia, PA: Hanley & Belfus; 2002:238–241.

Answers to the questions are located in Chapter 35.

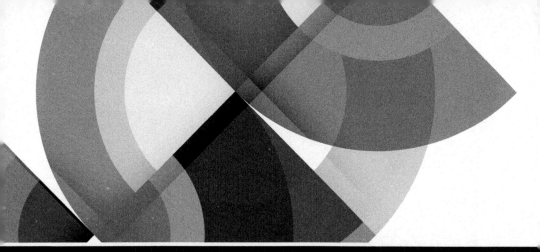

III NEEDLE EMG

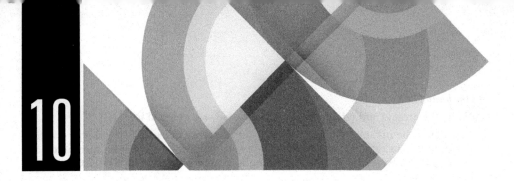

Basic EMG Technique

Christian M. Custodio

INTRODUCTION

Needle EMG is usually performed after nerve conduction studies have been completed, but can be performed first or by itself depending on the clinical indication. No electrical stimulation is used with EMG; the needle is simply a tool to measure the electrical activity in the muscle. The muscles that will be evaluated are chosen carefully based on the differential diagnosis. The examiner should evaluate only the minimum number of muscles that are necessary to do an adequate study, as examining more muscles may make the test more uncomfortable for the patient.

It is important to begin with an environment that is conducive to performing a study. Whenever possible, this includes a comfortable, quiet, interference-free environment, which is stocked with the appropriate supplies to limit interruptions.

PRESTUDY CHECKLIST

1. *At the patient:*
   - Introduce yourself, confirm the patient's identification, and verify the indication for the EMG (note: this may have been performed at the time of nerve conduction studies).
     - ☐ Give a brief overview of the test and reassure the patient about minimizing discomfort.
     - ☐ Ask about possible contraindications or precautions, such as anticoagulant use.
     - ☐ Verify the ground and reference electrode (if used) are in place.
     - ☐ The patient should be placed in a position of comfort.
     - ☐ The muscle being examined should be relaxed and accessible to the examiner.
     - ☐ Universal precautions (i.e., gloves) should be observed. Avoid examining areas of skin compromise such as open wounds, skin infections, or significant areas of edema or lymphedema.
     - ☐ Keep the patient covered everywhere at all times except the area being tested.
     - ☐ Ask for a chaperone when examining personal areas of any gender.
2. *At the EMG machine:*
   - Confirm that the gain, sweep speed, and filter settings are appropriate.

3. *At the preamplifier:*
   - Verify the ground and reference electrode (if used) are plugged in.
   - Make sure the preamplifier is turned on. To minimize noise and to prevent startling patients, it is recommended to insert the recording needle first before turning on the preamplifier. Likewise, turn off the preamplifier prior to removal of the EMG needle.
4. *Active electrode:*
   - The needle serves as the active electrode.
5. *Reference electrode:*
   - When a monopolar needle electrode is being used, a reference electrode is necessary. The reference should be near the location of needle insertion. If a concentric needle or single-fiber needle is used, a separate reference electrode is not necessary.

REDUCING ANXIETY AND DISCOMFORT OF THE NEEDLE EXAMINATION

Inform the patient before starting that some areas of the muscles may be uncomfortable. Instruct the patient to tell the examiner whether he or she is feeling discomfort so that the needle can be moved away from those areas. Pain is common if the needle is in the muscle end plate region. When this is apparent from the presence of end plate noise or spikes, quickly reposition the needle away from that area.

- Reassure the patient that almost everyone experiences some discomfort during the test, but most are able to tolerate it.
- Provide comfort and continued verbal sympathy with the patient throughout the study.
- Reassure the patient that any discomfort associated with the EMG is not long lasting.
- Insert the needle through the skin quickly, but move the needle within the muscle gently and slowly.
- Avoid hyperventilation.
- Patients may take pain medications prior to testing if they are concerned about the pain.
- Change needles if there is increased resistance or excessive pain associated with the needle movement.
- With especially anxious patients, begin with the most important muscle to minimize the number of needle insertions (e.g., paraspinal muscles in suspected radiculopathy).
- Warn the patient that some muscles (e.g., hand muscles or foot muscles) may be more sensitive than others.
- Reassure the patient that he or she can choose to discontinue the test at any time.

Clinical Pearl
- *Tip:* Evaluate each of the four basic components of standard EMG (insertional activity, spontaneous activity, motor unit analysis, and recruitment) for each muscle.

PROCEDURE PROTOCOL

1. Localize the muscle.
   - Find the muscle belly by using surface landmarks.
   - Confirm the position of the muscle belly itself. To do this, palpate the muscle belly and ask the patient to activate the muscle. The examiner should feel the muscle contraction.
   - Clean the area with an alcohol swab and let it dry.
   - Warn the patient before each new needle insertion.
2. Insert the needle.
   - Retract the skin making it taut, which helps the needle enter more easily.
   - In one quick motion, insert the needle tip through the skin into the subcutaneous tissue. Going slowly or softly increases discomfort.
   - If using a concentric needle, keeping the bevel side up during insertion will minimize discomfort.
   - Advance the needle through the subcutaneous tissue until the needle enters the muscle (Figure 10.1).

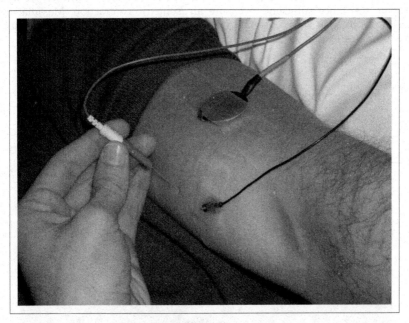

FIGURE 10.1 Needle electromyography.

3. Confirm the placement.
   - Once in the muscle tissue, ask the patient to slightly activate the muscle to confirm proper placement.
   - Provide sufficient resistance to ensure a gentle isometric contraction. If the needle is correctly placed, electrical activity will be seen on the screen and heard.

4. Evaluate insertional and spontaneous activity.
   - This is done by using the four-quadrant technique. In each quadrant do the following:
     - ☐ Advance the needle five times in a straight line. Each of these advancements should be small, 1 mm or less, to minimize patient discomfort.
     - ☐ Between each advancement, wait 1 to 2 seconds and listen for insertional and spontaneous activity.
     - ☐ Once five locations in the quadrant have been evaluated, slowly retract the needle until it is out of the muscle but remains in the subcutaneous tissue.
     - ☐ Adjust needle position and examine the next quadrant.
5. Analyze motor unit and evaluate recruitment.
   - *Isolation of a motor unit:* With the needle in the subcutaneous tissues, ask the patient to minimally activate the muscle being tested. Provide resistance sufficient to ensure an isometric contraction (Figure 10.2). Ask the patient to contract more or less to identify a predominant individual motor unit and to properly assess motor unit recruitment. Advance the needle into the muscle and adjust the needle to best analyze an individual motor unit potential. Do your calculations and record your findings (discussed later).
   - *Interference pattern:* Ask the patient to maximally activate the muscle being tested. Provide resistance sufficient to ensure an isometric contraction. Maximal intensity muscle contraction with a needle inserted can be very uncomfortable for patients, so this technique should be used sparingly.

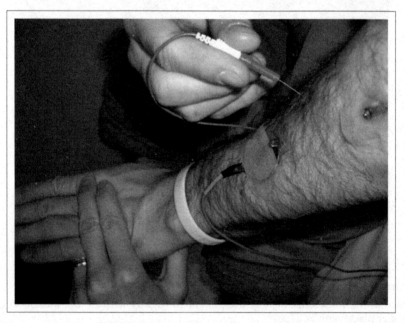

FIGURE 10.2 Isometric muscle contraction.

6. After each muscle is examined:
   - Remove the needle and apply local pressure with sterile gauze to achieve hemostasis after each muscle examined. Clean the area if necessary.
   - Ask the patient frequently how she or he is doing. Adjust your technique as necessary.
7. At completion of the study:
   - Dispose of the needle in a sharps container when finished.
   - Reassure the patient about his or her cooperation.
   - Sympathize with any discomfort.
   - Reassess the patient for areas of pain, bleeding, or bruising.
   - Ask whether the patient has any questions or concerns before leaving.
   - Describe the results of the test to the appropriate extent.

QUESTIONS

1. Which type of needle requires a reference electrode placed on the skin?
   A. Concentric
   B. Monopolar
   C. Single fiber

2. How many muscles are needed to complete an electromyogram study?
   A. 5
   B. 6
   C. The minimum needed to come to a conclusion
   D. The maximum the patient can tolerate

3. To minimize patient discomfort, what size needle movement is recommended?
   A. 1 mm
   B. 3 mm
   C. 5 mm
   D. 10 mm

ADDITIONAL READINGS

Daube JR. Assessing the motor unit with needle electromyography. In: Daube JR, ed. *Clinical Neurophysiology*. 2nd ed. New York, NY: Oxford University Press; 2002:293–323.

London ZN. Safety and pain in electrodiagnostic studies. *Muscle Nerve*. 2017;55:149–159. doi:10.1002/mus.25421

Strommen JA, Daube JR. Determinants of pain in needle electromyography. *Clin Neurophysiol*. 2001;112:1414–1418. PubMed PMID: 11459681.

Answers to the questions are located in Chapter 35.

Basic Approach to EMG Waveform Recognition

Gautam Malhotra and Chae K. Im

INTRODUCTION

EMG is a specific electrodiagnostic technique in which an electrode is used to visually and sonically display the electrical activity of muscle. The electromyographer usually inserts a needle electrode through the skin into specific muscles to acquire and display muscular electrical activity. The electromyographer is tasked with doing this while observing the evoked activity, identifying all waveforms, and interpreting their clinical significance "on the fly." The purpose of this chapter is to provide an approach to doing this with objective descriptions of various electrical activity that you will come across.

BASIC APPROACH

For the beginner, even observation can be challenging while trying to maneuver the needle. Although interpretation can be delayed until discussion with the instructor after the study, identification of waveforms must be done in real time as it occurs on the screen. This is a frustrating process if the trainee is not prepared with an approach; we present one here.

When performing needle EMG, the electrical activity seen on the screen can be broadly categorized as *insertion*, *voluntary*, or *spontaneous*.

1. **Insertion activity:** The electric activity caused by insertion or movement of a needle electrode within a muscle; that is, what you see on the screen because you moved the needle (Table 11.1).
2. **Voluntary activity:** Electric activity recorded from a muscle with consciously controlled contraction (Table 11.2).
3. **Spontaneous activity:** Electric activity recorded from a muscle at rest after insertion activity has subsided and when there is no voluntary activity; that is, the needle is not moving and the patient is completely relaxed (Tables 11.3 and 11.4).
4. **Artifact/other:** Noise from nearby equipment, pacemaker spikes, loose electrodes, faulty wires/cables, ringing cell phones, and so on.

Therefore, after ensuring a technically sound setup of equipment, the first step in identifying electrical activity is to decide within which category it belongs. This can usually be easily determined by paying close attention to what is happening to the needle and how relaxed

TABLE 11.1 Types of Insertion Activity and Their Attributes

Normal	Brief bursts of electrical potentials due to mechanical depolarization by the needle deforming the muscle membrane. Duration <300 ms.
Increased	Duration >300 ms, but <2–3 s. Any activity lasting longer should be reevaluated as possibly being voluntary or spontaneous. May reflect denervation or membrane instability.
Decreased	Little to no electrical activity with needle movement. First, ensure that the needle is in the correct location (easily done by asking the patient to contract the muscle)! Can be seen with fibrosis (i.e., connective tissue replacement of muscle), edema, and electrolyte abnormalities.

TABLE 11.2 Types of Voluntary Activity and Their Attributes

Motor unit action potential	• The summated electrical activity of muscle fibers innervated by a single axon. Only reflects those fibers within the range of the needle electrode. Amplitude usually reflects no more than 10 muscle fibers in the vicinity of the electrode while all of the muscle fibers belonging to the motor unit contribute to the duration. Usually triphasic. • Amplitude of 1st observed MUAPs ~300–500 µV. Later recruited MUAPs up to 3 mV. Giant refers to >5 mV • Duration: 5–15 ms. • Frequency: typically starts at 3–5 Hz and increases with effort up to >30 Hz. Not regular but "semirhythmic."
Polyphasic motor unit action potential	• Five or more phases. Up to 10% to 25% of recorded MUAPs may be polyphasic in normal muscles depending on the needle positioning. When pathologic, can be caused by collateral sprouting (seen with denervation) or dropout of muscle fibers (seen with myopathy).
MUAP, motor unit action potential.	

TABLE 11.3 Spontaneous Electrical Activity Originating in the Motor Neuron

Potential	Features	Origin and Conditions
Fasciculation potential (sporadic)	Same configuration as a single MUAP. Sporadic versus grouped. Sounds like a bird dropping against the windshield of a fast-moving car: "Thwack!"	Single, random, spontaneous twitch due to hyperirritation somewhere along the neuron, which activates all or a significant number of muscle fibers belonging to a single motor unit. Very often normal. Can also be grouped in pairs (doublets) or triplets.

(*continued*)

TABLE 11.3 Spontaneous Electrical Activity Originating in the Motor Neuron (*continued*)

Potential	Features	Origin and Conditions
Myokymic discharges (grouped fasciculations)	Same configuration as MUAP but two distinct firing patterns seen: 1. Brief uniform repetitive firing of MUAP at 40–60 Hz for up to a few seconds, with brief periods of interposed silence. Sounds like bursts of machine gun fire, or the drum solo from *One* by Metallica. 2. Continuous recurrent uniform slower firing 1–5 Hz. Sounds like "marching soldiers."	Originates somewhere along the motor neuron. Irregular discharge of motor unit possibly with ephaptic transmission. Sometimes seen with demyelinating conditions.
Neuromyotonic discharges	Abrupt start/stop. Fast (100–300 Hz) firing of single MUAP for few seconds. Progressive decrement/decrescendo (wanes). Characteristic "pinging" sound.	Rare. Burst of MUAPs originating at the motor axon. Seen in Isaac syndrome (neuromyotonia) and extremely chronic neuropathic diseases.
Cramp potentials	Same configuration as MUAP. Start and stop gradually. Can be very high frequency (up to 150 Hz). Slightly irregular.	Painful, involuntarily firing MUAPs originating in motor nerves. Can also be seen with fatigue or electrolyte imbalance.
MUAP, motor unit action potential.		

the patient appears to be. Most trainees understand this concept during their first electrodiagnostic encounter.

The fun begins when attempting to look for and identify spontaneous activity. Most of the time, one encounters silence at rest while the patient is relaxed. Spontaneous activity can be normal or abnormal depending on the observed behavior, constellation of findings, and clinical presentation. The attributes of many common spontaneous waveforms are included at the end of this section. Although memorizing their attributes and patterns is encouraged, **these should only be viewed as general guidelines**. There are unfortunately **no absolutes in EMG**. Any parameter can be wildly different in reality.

Upon initially learning how to read and interpret *electrocardiograms (ECG)*, pattern recognition can be a useful and appropriate technique. One would hope to apply this to EMG as well; however, this unfortunately becomes another common frustration for the in-training electromyographer. Certain waveforms can look and even behave exactly like other waveforms depending upon the screen settings (i.e., sensitivity and sweep speed), and the location of the needle electrode relative to the generated potential.

TABLE 11.4 Spontaneous Electrical Activity Originating in the Muscle Fiber

Name	Size	Duration	Frequency	Rhythm	Morphology	Sound	Conditions
Miniature end plate potential or "end plate noise"	Small (10–50 µV)	Short (0.5–2 ms)	Approx. every 5 s per axon terminal but clinically multiple observed at once	Irregular	Negative initial deflection; monophasic	Seashell murmur	Random, spontaneously released acetylcholine vesicles from nerve terminal at baseline elicit nonpropagating discharges at the muscle end plate.
End plate spikes	<300 µV	Short (2–4 ms)	50–100 Hz	Irregular	Biphasic with initial negative deflection	Sputtering fat in frying pan	Irritation by the needle electrode of the terminal axon results in a suprathreshold end plate depolarization of a single muscle fiber.
Fibrillation potentials (fibs) and positive sharp waves (Table 11.5)	<1 mV	Short (<5 ms)	Usually slow but wide range (1–50 Hz); often decreases just before cessation	Usually regular	Biphasic with initial positive deflection	"Rain on a tin roof"; ticking. PSW: Dull thud	Fibs are generated by one single physiologically unstable sarcolemma. The resting membrane potential slowly creeps upward until the threshold is reached; a spontaneous depolarization occurs, followed by repolarization, with the cycle beginning over again. PSW are thought to be a variation of the fibrillation except that the muscle fiber at the recording site is deformed by the presence of the needle electrode. The unstable resting membrane potential leading to fibrillation potentials and PSW can occur from direct muscle injury (trauma, inflammation) or denervation.

(continued)

TABLE 11.4 Spontaneous Electrical Activity Originating in the Muscle Fiber (*continued*)

Name	Size	Duration	Frequency	Rhythm	Morphology	Sound	Conditions
Complex repetitive discharge (aka bizarre repetitive discharges, pseudomyotonia)	<1 mV	Variable, but start/stop abruptly	0.3–150 Hz	Regular	May display abrupt changes in configuration	Machinery	• Group of single muscle fibers spontaneously depolarizing in a set pattern directed by a primary pacemaker fiber. • Usually seen in chronic processes in which a group of muscle fibers become unstable similar to those of fibs and PSW (denervation, myopathy). • May also be normally seen in iliopsoas muscle.
Myotonic discharges	10 μV–1 mV	>5–20 ms	20–100 Hz	Waxing and waning	Waxing and waning amplitude and frequency	WWII dive bomber; intermittently accelerated, idling motorcycle	Rapid, repetitive, variable waxing/waning in amplitude and frequent firing of fibs or PSW-appearing potentials. The primary defect is in the membrane's ionic conductance characteristics. Requires needle movement or muscle contraction.

PSW, positive sharp waves.

TABLE 11.5 Grading of Positive Sharp Wave and Fibrillation Potential Activity

Grade	Meaning
0	None present
+1	Fibrillation potentials persistent in at least two areas
+2	Moderate number of persistent fibrillation potentials in three or more areas
+3	Large number of persistent discharges in all areas
+4	Profuse, widespread, persistent discharges that fill the baseline

Source: Adapted from Daube JR, Rubin DI. Needle electromyography. *Muscle Nerve.* 2009;39(2):244–270. doi:10.1002/mus.21180

QUESTIONS

1. Which of the following potentials originates prejunctionally?
   A. Fasciculation potentials
   B. Fibrillation potentials
   C. Myotonic discharges
   D. Positive sharp waves

2. Which normal spontaneous potential is typically confused with fibrillation potentials?
   A. Fasciculation potentials
   B. End plate spikes
   C. Voluntary motor unit action potential
   D. Positive sharp waves

3. Which of the following potentials originates postjunctionally?
   A. Fasciculation potentials
   B. Myokymic discharges
   C. Myotonic discharges
   D. Neuromyotonic discharges

4. Which of the following potentials is thought to be generated by a pacemaker muscle fiber and ephaptic transmission to neighboring muscle fibers?
   A. Fasciculation potentials
   B. Complex repetitive discharges
   C. Myotonic discharges
   D. Myokymic discharges

Answers to the questions are located in Chapter 35.

ADDITIONAL READINGS

American Association of Electrodiagnostic Medicine. *AAEM Glossary of Terms in Electrodiagnostic Medicine. Muscle and Nerve*. Rochester, MN: American Association of Electrodiagnostic Medicine; 2001.

Daube JR, Rubin DI. Needle electromyography. *Muscle Nerve*. 2009;39(2):244–270. doi:10.1002/mus.21180

Dumitru D, Zwarts MJ. Needle electromyography. In: Dumitru D, Amato A, Zwarts MJ, eds. *Electrodiagnostic Medicine*. Philadelphia, PA: Hanley & Belfus; 2002:chap 7.

Preston DC, Shapiro BE. In: Basic electromyography: analysis of motor unit action potentials. *Electromyography and Neuromuscular Disorders: Clinical-Electrophysiologic Correlations*. Philadelphia, PA: Butterworth-Heinemann; 2005:chap15.

12

Motor Unit Action Potential Analysis

Anirudh Gupta, Kasser Saba, and W. David Arnold

INTRODUCTION

- A motor unit consists of a single motor neuron and all the muscle fibers it innervates.
- The number of muscle fibers innervated per motor neuron is referred to as the *innervation ratio*.
- Innervation ratio varies depending on muscle size: Muscles that are used for precise movements generally have smaller innervation ratios.

OVERVIEW OF THE MOTOR UNIT ACTION POTENTIAL

- A motor unit action potential (MUAP) is the EMG response that results from the discharge of all the muscle fibers that are innervated by a single motor neuron.
- An MUAP, therefore, represents the summation potential of all of the muscle fiber action potentials (APs) that are elicited by their common motor neuron and that are close enough to the tip of the recording electrode to be able to be registered.
- The size and shape of MUAPs are dependent on the size, number, and functional state of muscle fibers innervated by a single motor neuron (in the region of the recording electrode).
- The size and shape of an MUAP can be described in terms of amplitude, duration, phasicity, and stability.
- In the healthy state, an MUAP is stable due to the all-or-none nature of APs as well as the reliability of neuromuscular transmission (i.e., safety factor).
- Denervation, dysfunction of the neuromuscular junction transmission, or altered excitability of muscle fibers may cause MUAPs to become unstable, that is, having variable sizes and shapes between consecutive discharges.
- Firing characteristics and recruitment of motor units can also be quantified, enabling identification of different patterns of pathology of the neuromuscular system.

MOTOR UNIT MORPHOLOGY
Duration
- The duration of an MUAP is the total amount of time of the recorded potential and is measured from the initial deflection from the baseline potential until the final return to baseline potential (Figure 12.1).
- MUAP duration correlates with the number of muscle fibers that are innervated by a single motor neuron in the region of the recording electrode.
- During processes of muscle fiber degeneration or inexcitability, the MUAP duration will be shortened.
- During processes of denervation, collateral sprouting, and reinnervation, increased numbers of muscle fibers will be innervated by a single motor neuron in the region of the recording electrode (i.e., grouped reinnervation) leading to increased MUAP duration.
- Reference values for MUAP duration are between 5 and 15 ms.

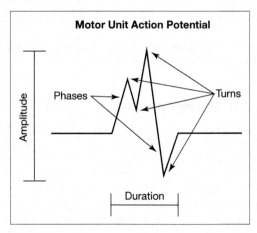

FIGURE 12.1 Representative motor unit action potential demonstrating the parameters of amplitude, duration, phasicity, and turns.

Amplitude
- MUAP amplitude is generally measured from the maximal negative peak to the maximal positive peak of the MUAP (Figure 12.1).
- The amplitude of an MUAP reflects the number of muscle fibers innervated by a single motor neuron (in the region of the recording electrode).
- Amplitude of an MUAP is also influenced by the size of individual muscle fibers closest to the recording electrode. Therefore, MUAP amplitude is less well correlated with the numbers of muscle fibers innervated by a motor neuron.
- Reference values for MUAP amplitudes are related to electrode type.
- The normal amplitude for most MUAPs is between 100 µV and 2 mV. An upper limit of 6 mV is generally used for a monopolar electrode and 4 mV for a concentric electrode.

Phasicity
- The term "phase" is used to describe the individual components of an MUAP that are above and below the baseline. In Figure 12.1, a representative MUAP is shown with two phases.
- The number of phases in an MUAP can be calculated by taking the number of baseline crossings and adding 1 (e.g., in Figure 12.1 this would be 1 + 1 = 2).
- The term "turn" describes a change in amplitude of the MUAP that does not cross the baseline.
- Most MUAPs will have between two and four phases. MUAPs with greater than four phases are referred to as being *polyphasic*.
- Polyphasia is the result of desynchronization of the summation of the muscle fiber AP that contribute to an MUAP.
- Desynchronization can occur due to early reinnervation as well as degeneration and regeneration of muscle fibers. Thus, polyphasic MUAPs are nonspecific.
- A percentage of MUAPs within a healthy muscle will be polyphasic.

Stability
- An MUAP represents the summated muscle fiber APs within the recording area of the needle electrode that are innervated by a single motor neuron.
- In the healthy state, due to both the all-or-none phenomenon of muscle fiber APs and the reliability of neuromuscular junction transmission, the MUAP potential size does not vary between discharges and is completely stable.
- If changes in MUAP size and shape are observed in a healthy patient, it is most likely related to movement of either the needle electrode or the muscle.
- In contrast, pathological changes—such as abnormal neuromuscular junction transmission or abnormal excitability of muscle fibers—can result in variability of MUAP size and shape between consecutive discharges.

CHANGES IN MUAP CHARACTERISTICS AND MORPHOLOGY IN DISEASE
Myopathies
- Short-duration, small amplitude, and polyphasic MUAPs are characteristic of myopathic processes.
- A variety of myopathic processes can result in disruption of muscle fiber AP generation. Some of these may include immune cell invasion of muscle fibers (inflammatory myopathies such as dermatomyositis), necrosis of muscle fibers (immune processes, toxic exposure, others), and inexcitability (such as periodic paralysis).
- Loss of muscle fiber integrity or function may result in loss of muscle fiber AP generation.
- Losses of muscle fiber AP result in a reduced size of the summated MUAP amplitude during an EMG recording of a myopathic muscle.
- In the cases of very chronic myopathies characterized by cycles of degeneration and regeneration of muscle fibers (such as milder forms of muscular dystrophy or inclusion body myositis), MUAPs may become complex and polyphasic in appearance.

- MUAP amplitudes are generally reduced in myopathies, because of a reduced number and/or excitability of muscle fibers. However, chronic myopathies can display muscle fiber hypertrophy, which in turn can lead to MUAPs with increased amplitude.
- Increased MUAP amplitude in myopathic conditions usually reflects muscle fiber hypertrophy rather than grouped reinnervation (i.e., increased numbers of muscle fibers being innervated by the same single motor neuron in the region of the recording electrode).

Denervation and Reinnervation (Collateral Sprouting and Axonal Regeneration)

- Long-duration, large amplitude, polyphasic MUAPs are characteristic of neuropathic processes.
- Denervation leads to a reduction in the number of motor neurons/units that are functionally connected to a particular muscle.
- In the acute setting (up to 8 weeks), this, however, does not usually result in immediate changes in MUAP size or shape.
- Denervated muscle fibers can be reinnervated through mechanisms of either (i) collateral sprouting or (ii) axonal regeneration.
- Collateral sprouting occurs when denervation is partial or incomplete; terminal axons of motor units that are intact "sprout" (and hence "expand") to reconnect to denervated muscle fibers.
- Following collateral reinnervation, a single motor neuron will have increased the number of muscle fibers it innervates (in the region of the recording electrode); the resulting MUAP will be increased in size (both amplitude and duration).
- As it takes time for these new axon collateral sprouts and neuromuscular junctions to mature, MUAPs during the early stages of reinnervation will have increased polyphasia.
- MUAP changes in collateral sprouting are usually noted approximately 8 weeks following partial denervation.
- In contrast to collateral sprouting, axonal regeneration is a delayed phenomenon dependent on axonal regrowth from the site of nerve injury toward the denervated target muscle.
- During axonal regeneration, the first synaptic connections made with a denervated muscle will be with only a few muscle fibers resulting in MUAPs of reduced size.
- These early, small, immature MUAPs that result from axonal regeneration are sometimes referred to as *nascent* MUAPs.
- Over time, these new, nascent MUAPs can become larger (amplitude and duration) as more muscle fibers are reinnervated.
- In contrast to collateral sprouting, which is reliably evident within approximately 8 weeks, the efficacy and timing of axonal regeneration is dependent on the distance of the target muscle from the site of nerve injury.
- Longer distances between the target muscle and the site of injury result in longer duration prior to reinnervation as well as less effective reinnervation.

QUESTIONS

1. Motor unit action potential (MUAP) duration is best correlated with which anatomical factor?
   A. Muscle fiber size
   B. Number of motor units connected to a muscle within the recording area of the needle electrode
   C. Number of muscle fibers innervated by a motor neuron (innervation ratio)
   D. Number of muscle fibers innervated by a motor neuron within the recording area of the needle electrode

2. A resident is performing an evaluation of the motor units in the biceps of a patient with weakness. She notes motor unit action potentials (MUAPs) with amplitudes of 7 mV, duration of 25 ms, and five or more phases. Which of the following is a true statement?
   A. These are normal MUAPs.
   B. These are abnormal MUAPs, likely due to acute denervation.
   C. These are abnormal MUAPs, likely due to denervation without reinnervation.
   D. These are abnormal MUAPs, likely due to denervation with reinnervation.
   E. None of the above.

3. A 55-year-old woman presents with symmetric, proximal limb weakness and a rash that has progressed over the last 6 months. The patient is suspected to have dermatomyositis. During EMG recordings you expect to see which of the following?
   A. Decreased MUAP amplitude
   B. Decreased MUAP duration
   C. Polyphasic MUAPs
   D. Both A and B
   E. A, B, C

4. A 33-year-old man is seen in follow-up for a history of right upper limb weakness related to Parsonage–Turner syndrome that affected his axillary nerve. His prior EMG study 1 month after symptom onset showed abnormal spontaneous activity (active denervation) and no motor unit action potentials (MUAPs) being recruited in his right deltoid muscle. Today, 6 months after his symptom onset, a repeat EMG study is performed. Clinical examination demonstrates possible slight muscle twitches in his deltoid muscle when the patient attempts maximally to abduct his right shoulder. During EMG recordings of his right deltoid muscle during maximal shoulder abduction, three discrete polyphasic MUAPs with shortened durations (<5 ms) are observed. Which of the following is true regarding this finding?
   A. The short duration of the MUAPs is related to degeneration of muscle fibers.
   B. The short duration of the MUAPs is related to early axonal sprouting.
   C. The polyphasia of the MUAPs is related to increased numbers of muscle fibers innervated by the same motor unit due to collateral sprouting.
   D. The short duration of the MUAPs is related to collateral sprouting.
   E. None of the above.

Answers to the questions are located in Chapter 35.

13

Recruitment

Monal Desai and W. David Arnold

INTRODUCTION

- *Motor unit recruitment* refers to the sequential activation of motor units during an increasing muscle contraction (Figure 13.1).
- Recruitment is one of the main aspects of motor unit action potential (MUAP) analysis during the needle EMG examination.
- Recruitment can be used to distinguish normal versus underlying myopathic or neuropathic conditions (Figure 13.2).

OVERVIEW OF RECRUITMENT

- During muscle contraction, force output is modulated by the number of motor units recruited and the rate of motor unit discharge.
- Under voluntary control, motor neurons and motor units fire semirhythmically and no slower than 4 to 5 Hz. During normal contractions the maximal motor unit firing rates are usually less than 50 Hz, but during ballistic contractions firing rates of motor units may reach over 100 Hz.
- According to the size principle, during gradually increasing muscle contractions, smaller motor units (innervating type I muscle fibers) are recruited first followed by larger motor units (innervating type II muscle fibers).

BASICS OF RECRUITMENT ANALYSIS

- Recruitment is particularly helpful in identifying disorders of the peripheral nervous system.
- Simply stated, recruitment is assessed by determining whether the MUAPs activated during a muscle contraction are firing at appropriate rates.
- MUAP recruitment is best evaluated at minimal to moderate levels of muscle contraction to allow discernment of individual MUAPs.
- Recruitment pattern can be described as normal, early (increased; seen in myopathic conditions), or late (decreased; seen in neuropathic conditions).
- Recruitment can be quantified using recruitment ratio (see Table 13.1 for calculations).

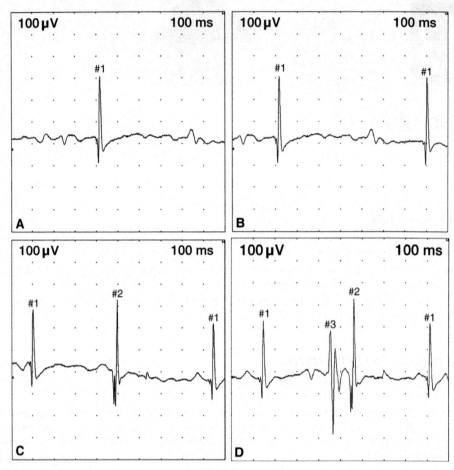

FIGURE 13.1 Normal recruitment of three MUAPs during concentric needle electromyography of a muscle during a gradually increasing contraction. MUAPs are labeled #1 to #3 in the order of recruitment. (A) Single MUAP. (B) Single MUAP now firing at a faster rate. (C) An additional MUAP is recruited. (D) A 3rd MUAP is recruited.

MUAP, motor unit action potential.

- Normal recruitment is characterized by a normal number of recruited motor units firing at a normal rate (and therefore normal recruitment ratio).
- Neuropathic conditions result in late (or reduced) recruitment with reduced number of motor units firing at higher frequencies (i.e., high recruitment ratio).
- Myopathic conditions result in early (or increased) recruitment with increased numbers of motor units recruited than would be expected for the amount of force produced during a muscle contraction.
- Recruitment is not altered in upper motor neuron pathology.
- In upper motor neuron disorders or insufficient patient effort, activation of motor units may be reduced, resulting in reduced numbers of motor units firing at low frequencies.

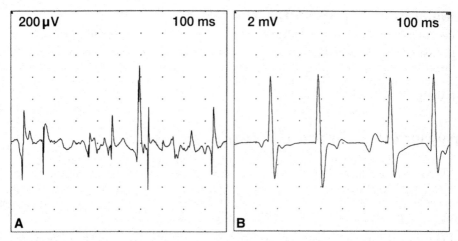

FIGURE 13.2 Abnormal patterns of MUAP recruitment. (A) Early recruitment and short duration MUAPs in a patient with inclusion body myositis providing a weak muscle contraction. (B) Late (reduced) recruitment in a patient with chronic motor neuron disease, displaying a large amplitude MUAP with a firing rate of approximately 40 Hz.

MUAP, motor unit action potential.

TABLE 13.1 Quantitative Recruitment Parameters

Calculation of Firing Rate (Examples Using Figure 13.1D)
1. Determine how many screens there are in 1 s. *Example using Figure 13.1B:* *Screen-sweep speed equals 100 ms (10 ms/div)* *1000 ms/100 ms = 10 screens in 1 second*
2. Count how many times an individual MUAP appears on the screen. *The fastest firing MUAP is seen twice on the 100 ms screen.*
3. Multiply the number of screens in a second by the number of occurrences of the particular MUAP to determine firing rate. *Firing rate = 2 × 10 = 20 Hz*
Calculation of Recruitment Ratio (Examples Using Figure 13.1D)
1. Calculate firing rate of fastest MUAP. *Example using Figure 13.1B:* *As calculated earlier, the fastest firing MUAP is seen twice per screen and the number of screens in 1 s is 10. Therefore, the firing rate of the MUAP is 20 Hz.*
2. Count total number of MUAPs on screen. *Total number of MUAPS = 3. A total of three distinct MUAPs are seen.*
3. Divide firing rate by total number of MUAP. *Recruitment ratio = 20/3 = ~7.*
MUAP, motor unit action potential.

CLINICAL UTILITY OF RECRUITMENT ANALYSIS
- Recruitment analysis can help identify a myopathic versus a neuropathic process.
- Decreased recruitment may be present immediately following axonal injury or dysfunction; therefore, decreased recruitment is an early finding as compared with other findings such as MUAP morphological changes or membrane stability (i.e., abnormal spontaneous activity).

STEPWISE APPROACH TO RECRUITMENT ASSESSMENT
1. Confirm that the gain and sweep-speed settings are appropriate to fully view the MUAPs and to allow recruitment quantification. Sensitivity setting will depend on the size of the MUAPs and should be set to allow full visualization of the MUAPs. Sweep speed is somewhat dependent on personal preference, but is usually set at 100 or 200 ms.
2. Based on the differential diagnosis, determine the muscles to be tested.
3. Place the patient in a position that facilitates isometric contraction and have the patient perform a minimal to moderate contraction to allow visualization and analysis of discrete MUAPs.
4. To assess recruitment, the number and the firing rates of the MUAPs present in a contraction muscle need to be determined. Newer electrodiagnostic devices allow storage of EMG signals for review after completion of a muscle assessment. This can be a particularly helpful feature for less experienced electromyographers.
5. Distinct MUAPs are identified and quantified based on different waveform shapes (see Figures 13.1 and 13.2).
6. To calculate the firing rate of an MUAP, simply determine how many times the MUAP is seen within a span of 1 second (e.g., if the sweep speed of the screen is set at 200 ms, multiply the number of MUAP occurrences by 5; if the sweep speed is set at 100 ms, multiply the number of MUAP occurrences by 10).

MAXIMAL ACTIVATION-INTERFERENCE PATTERN
- The confluence of motor units that appear on the screen with maximal muscle activation is known as the *interference pattern*.
- For a normal healthy muscle with intact motor unit innervation, maximal contraction results in MUAPs filling the screen. Performing maximal contraction in a healthy muscle with intact innervation usually does not provide valuable information and can be painful for patients.
- With neuropathic processes, loss of motor units will result in reduced interference (sometimes referred to as a *picket fence pattern*).
- For myopathic processes, the interference pattern may fill up the screen (assuming there isn't severe muscle loss), but the MUAPs will be reduced in size.

TABLE 13.2 Expected Recruitment Findings

	Normal	Acute Motor Axonal Loss or Conduction Block	Chronic Motor Axonal Loss	Myopathy	Upper Motor Neuron Weakness
Recruitment	Normal	Late (decreased)	Late to normal recruitment (depending on the recovery of a normal number of innervating axons)	Early (increased)	Normal
Recruitment ratio	Normal (5–<10:1)	Increased (>10:1)	Increased to normal depending on the level of recovery	Normal (5–<10:1)	Normal (5–<10:1)
Maximal activation Interference Pattern	Full	Decreased number of MUAPs firing at high rates (i.e., picket fence pattern)	Decreased to full Depends on the level of reinnervation, but may have decreased the number of units with picket fence appearance of larger polyphasic MUAPs	Full In chronic myopathies severe muscle degeneration can result in dropout of MUAPs and decreased interference	Few, slowly firing MUAPs (i.e., decreased activation)

MUAP, motor unit action potential.

RECRUITMENT FINDINGS IN NEUROPATHIC PROCESSES

- In neuropathic processes, loss of MUAPs on the needle electrode examination may be the result of either conduction block or axonal loss. The remaining MUAPs recruited during a muscle contraction will be firing at a higher than expected rate (Table 13.2).
- In the case of a chronic axonal nerve injury, recruitment may normalize if the motor units are able to reestablish normal innervation patterns via axonal sprouting. In contrast, collateral sprouting will not correct reduced or late recruitment following axonal injury (although MUAP size will increase in amplitude and duration due to increased numbers of muscles fibers innervated by a single motor neuron).

RECRUITMENT FINDINGS IN MYOPATHIC PROCESSES

- In myopathic processes, muscle fibers undergo degeneration. Therefore, each motor unit produces a reduced force output during muscle contraction.
- For a given level of contraction in a myopathic muscle, an increased number of MUAPs will be recruited (i.e., early/increased recruitment) out of proportion for the resultant muscle force.

QUESTIONS

1. What is the firing rate of an MUAP that is seen five times on a screen with a sweep speed set at 20 ms/div with a total of 10 divisions on the screen?
   A. 4 Hz
   B. 25 Hz
   C. 50 Hz
   D. 100 Hz

2. You have been asked to perform an EMG examination on a patient who suffered a partial right upper trunk brachial plexus injury 2 weeks ago. During the examination of his right biceps brachii muscle, what would you expect his recruitment ratio to be?
   A. Normal
   B. Increased
   C. Decreased
   D. No recruitment

3. When performing a needle EMG study, a single voluntary MUAP appears per sweep speed on the screen and slowly moves toward the right. With the sweep speed set at 10 ms/div (10 divisions on the screen), what is the frequency of the potential?
   A. 8 Hz
   B. 10 Hz
   C. 12 Hz
   D. 20 Hz

4. When performing a needle EMG study, on maximal muscle activation the interference pattern in an acute neuropathic process would most likely show:
   A. Full interference
   B. Delayed interference
   C. Picket fence appearance on the screen
   D. Screen filled with large motor units that are large and polyphasic.

Answers to the questions are located in Chapter 35.

ADDITIONAL READINGS

American Association of Electrodiagnostic Medicine. Glossary of terms in clinical electromyography. *Muscle Nerve.* 2001;24(suppl):10. doi:10.1002/mus.1188

Duabe JR, Rubin DI. Needle electromyography. *Muscle Nerve.* 2009;39:244–270. doi:10.1002/mus.21180

Dumitru D, Zwarts MJ. Needle electromyography. In: Dumitru D, Amato AA, Zwarts MJ, eds. *Electrodiagnostic Medicine.* 2nd ed. Philadelphia, PA: Hanley & Belfus; 2002:257–291.

Preston DC, Shapiro BE. Basic electromyography: analysis of motor unit action potentials. In: Preston DC, Shapiro BE, eds. *Electromyography and Neuromuscular Disorders: Clinical-Electrophysiologic Correlations.* Boston, MA: Butterworth-Heinemann; 1998:191–205.

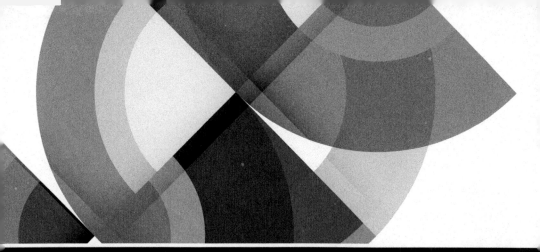

IV IMPORTANT CONCEPTS FOR INTERPRETING STUDIES

14

Orthodromic and Antidromic Nerve Conduction Studies

Daniel A. Goodman

INTRODUCTION

- **Physiologic nerve conduction**
    - Nerve conduction studies (NCS) typically involve mixed nerves, such that they include both sensory and motor nerve fibers.
    - Motor nerve action potentials propagate from the anterior horn cell distally toward the neuromuscular junction.
    - Sensory nerve action potentials (SNAP) propagate from the sensory nerve endings proximally toward the dorsal root ganglion.
- **Conduction during NCS**
    - Propagation of an induced action potential during NCS travels in both directions, proximally and distally.
    - In an **orthodromic** study, the recording electrodes measure the action potential traveling in the physiologic direction.
    - In an **antidromic** study, the recording electrodes measure the action potential traveling opposite the physiologic direction.
    - All motor NCS are orthodromic.
    - Sensory NCS can be either orthodromic or antidromic.
    - Conduction velocities and latencies are equal in both directions (1–3).
    - Antidromic SNAP amplitudes are larger than orthodromic SNAP amplitudes. This phenomenon is attributed to the more superficial course of the sensory nerves distally such that the recording electrode is in closer proximity to the signal generated. Other explanations for the reduced amplitude of orthodromic sensory NCS are that the distal branches of the nerves are thinner and/or less excitable (2,3).

MOTOR NERVE CONDUCTION STUDIES

- These orthodromic studies measure the compound motor action potential (CMAP) in the physiologic direction, such that the stimulation site is proximal and the recording electrode is placed distally over the muscle belly.

SENSORY NERVE CONDUCTION STUDIES

- Sensory nerve studies can be performed antidromically or orthodromically.
- During antidromic recordings, the nerve is stimulated proximally and the recording electrode is placed distally (Figure 14.1).
- During orthodromic recordings, the sensory nerve is stimulated distally and the recording electrode is placed proximally (Figure 14.2).
- One of the most clinically relevant assessments that utilizes both orthodromic and antidromic sensory NCS is the combined sensory index (CSI) for the median nerve (see Chapter 18). The CSI utilizes a comparison of the median and ulnar nerve latencies in which the antidromic study is recorded at the 4th digit and stimulated over each nerve proximally and the orthodromic study is recorded over the proximal respective nerve and stimulated at the midpalm (2).

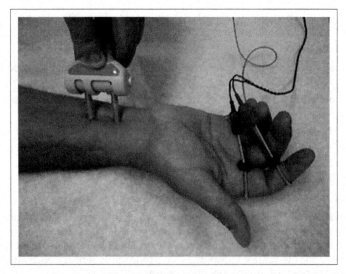

FIGURE 14.1 Antidromic median sensory nerve conduction study electrode and stimulator placement.

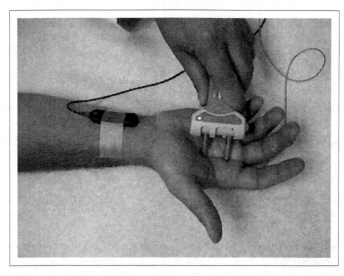

FIGURE 14.2 Orthodromic median sensory nerve conduction study electrode and stimulator placement.

CONSIDERATIONS FOR SENSORY NERVE CONDUCTION STUDIES

- The higher amplitudes observed in antidromic studies are considered an advantage. There is, nevertheless, a potential disadvantage of antidromic studies as proximal stimulation is usually performed over a mixed nerve where both sensory and motor fibers are stimulated (2). The motor stimulation may induce a CMAP recording. An inexperienced practitioner may confuse this CMAP for a SNAP. This phenomenon can be more problematic when the distal latency of the SNAP is prolonged. Because motor nerves are not usually stimulated in orthodromic sensory NCS, recording of a CMAP is not a problem.
- Anatomical variation, such as digit or limb size, can contribute to amplitude differences. The amplitude of the median SNAP in both orthodromic and antidromic studies has been shown to be inversely proportional to wrist thickness (2). The amplitude of both median and ulnar antidromic NCS is inversely proportional to finger circumference (2,3).

QUESTIONS

1. When performing an H-reflex, the M-wave represents a signal equivalent to which type of NCS?
   A. Orthodromic motor NCS
   B. Antidromic NCS
   C. Orthodromic sensory NCS
   D. Nonphysiologic response

Answers to the questions are located in Chapter 35.

2. In order to avoid recording a motor action potential during a sensory NCS, the signal should be obtaining using which type of study?
   A. H-reflex at supramaximal stimulation
   B. Orthodromic sensory NCS
   C. Antidromic sensory NCS
   D. Orthodromic motor NCS

3. The action potential generated during a motor nerve NCS travels in which direction?
   A. Orthodromic direction only
   B. Antidromic direction only
   C. Both physiologic and nonphysiologic directions
   D. Variable depending on temperature

4. The combined sensory index (CSI) for evaluation of median mononeuropathy at the wrist uses which NCS studies?
   A. Orthodromic motor NCS only
   B. Antidromic and orthodromic motor NCS
   C. Antidromic and orthodromic sensory NCS
   D. Orthodromic sensory NCS only

REFERENCES

1. Buchthal F, Rosenfalck A. Evoked action potentials and conduction velocity in human sensory nerves. *Brain Res.* 1966;9:1–122. doi:10.1016/0006-8993(66)90056-4
2. Valls-Sole J, Leote J, Pereira P. Antidromic vs orthodromic sensory median nerve conduction studies. *Clin Neurophysiol Pract.* 2016;1:18–25. doi:10.1016/j.cnp.2016.02.004
3. Gentili G, Di Napoli M. Wrist, elbow—digit IV, V; wrist—digit IV, V. In: Gentili G, Di Napoli M, eds. *The Ulnar Nerve*. Basel, Switzerland: Springer International Publishing; 2016:33–43.

Temporal Dispersion and Phase Cancellation

Mary Ann Miknevich and Jenna Meriggi

INTRODUCTION

Phase cancellation and temporal dispersion are vital concepts for the electromyographer to understand in order to accurately interpret variations in recorded compound potentials (sensory nerve action potentials [SNAPs,], compound muscle action potentials [CMAPs]) that are seen with distal and proximal stimulation. This becomes important in determining physiologic from pathologic conditions.

Although the concepts are intrinsically linked and represent the same underlying electrophysiological principle, the best way to begin understanding them is by first separating them.

BASIC CONCEPTS

- Evoked potentials recorded in standard nerve conduction studies are a response summation of electrical fields produced by depolarization along nerve and muscle fibers of varying size.
- The muscle fiber is the source of the CMAP in motor conductions.
- The nerve axon is the source of the SNAP.
- Large fibers depolarize more quickly (faster) than small fibers (slower).
- During a motor and sensory nerve conduction study, stimulating a nerve at both proximal and distal sites while recording from a single location (recording electrode site) produces waveforms with slight differences in morphology.
- The potential closest to the recording electrode (distal stimulation site) will be larger in amplitude and shorter in duration. The potential farthest from the recording electrode (proximal stimulation site) will be smaller in amplitude and longer in duration.
- This is a normal phenomenon, known as *temporal dispersion,* which occurs because there will be a difference in the conduction speeds of different fibers.
  - Temporal dispersion is the increase in the difference between the conduction times along the different axons within a nerve (1,2). With increased distance, there is a larger difference in the times of arrival between the fastest and slowest conducting nerve fibers.

Area under the curve

- Area under the curve (AUC) is the negative peak amplitude (height) × negative peak duration (length) of a potential. This equals the summation of all potentials (axons) for a given compounded potential (see Table 15.1).
- If potentials arrive at the recording electrode at the same time, the greater the summation will be and, therefore, the greater the amplitude.
- If potentials arrive separately, the greater the duration.
- Assuming a constant AUC (i.e., same number of axons stimulated with each recording) yields an inverse ratio between duration and amplitude. AUC = amplitude × duration. In other words, if duration increases, amplitude decreases proportionately and vice versa.

TABLE 15.1 The Race Analogy

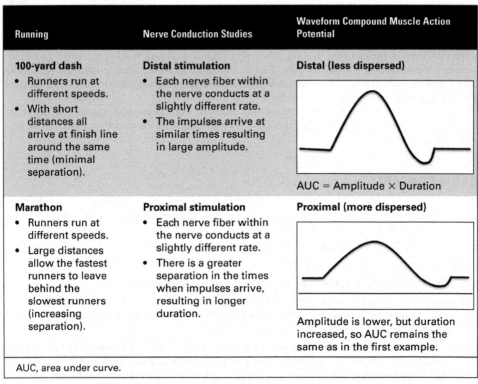

Running	Nerve Conduction Studies	Waveform Compound Muscle Action Potential
100-yard dash • Runners run at different speeds. • With short distances all arrive at finish line around the same time (minimal separation).	**Distal stimulation** • Each nerve fiber within the nerve conducts at a slightly different rate. • The impulses arrive at similar times resulting in large amplitude.	**Distal (less dispersed)** AUC = Amplitude × Duration
Marathon • Runners run at different speeds. • Large distances allow the fastest runners to leave behind the slowest runners (increasing separation).	**Proximal stimulation** • Each nerve fiber within the nerve conducts at a slightly different rate. • There is a greater separation in the times when impulses arrive, resulting in longer duration.	**Proximal (more dispersed)** Amplitude is lower, but duration increased, so AUC remains the same as in the first example.

AUC, area under curve.

- **Summated overall potential seen during a nerve conduction study** = the sum of upward (negative) potentials − the sum of downward (positive) potentials.
- The distance between two impulses traveling at different speeds will be larger with increased time.
  - This can be explained with the example of runners running a 100-yard dash, compared to those in a marathon, as listed in Table 15.1.
  - In both scenarios, AUC is preserved. The total number of axons arriving at the recording electrode is the same.
- Although present in both SNAPs and CMAPs, the decrease in amplitude and increase in duration seen with proximal compared to distal stimulation is most evident and usually noted in sensory conductions.
  - This is due to a combination of temporal dispersion as well as a principle known as *phase cancellation*.
- **Phase cancellation is the cancellation of part of an evoked potential produced by the overlap of positive and negative components.**
  - Action potentials have both negative upward deflections and positive downward deflections. If individual potentials arrive at the same time (in **synchrony**) so that all the upward deflections line up and all the downward deflections line up, the result would be a large negative (upward deflection) followed by a large positive (downward) deflection.
  - With longer distances, when there is more time for separation, the potentials would not line up but rather spread apart from each other and increase the duration. In this case, asynchronous axon potentials occur, such that the negative deflection of one potential now arrives at the same time as the positive deflection of another potential. The upward and downward phases tend to negate each other.
  - Because routine nerve conduction values only display the final summation, cancelled potentials appear as never having arrived at the recording electrode even though they did.
  - In this situation, despite increased duration, the amplitude is artificially decreased even further than would normally occur, resulting in an artificially low AUC.
  - It would be tempting to read the results as pathological because the amplitude drop was not accompanied by a proportional increase in duration, but the actual number of axons arriving at the recording electrode is preserved and the loss of AUC is nothing more than a mathematical construct.
  - Slight latency differences in SNAPs can cause the negative peaks of slower fibers to coincide with the positive peaks of faster fibers, leading to up to a 50% reduction in SNAP area and amplitude.
  - Less effect is noted with CMAPs as they are of longer duration and less phase cancellation occurs as they tend to superimpose more closely in phase over the same latency difference.
- An example of phase cancellation is listed in Table 15.2.

TABLE 15.2 Continuing the Race Analogy

Running	Nerve Conduction Studies	Waveform Compound Muscle Action Potential
	Distal stimulation	**Distal (less dispersed)**
• Runners A, B, and C challenge each other to a race. • With short distances all arrive at the finish line around the same time (minimal separation).	• Each nerve fiber within the nerve conducts at a slightly different rate. • The impulses arrive at similar times resulting in large amplitude.	A B C
Marathon	**Proximal stimulation**	**Proximal (more dispersed)**
• Runner A extends his lead and runner B slightly overtakes runner C. • However, runner C is now completely masked from a sideline observer by runner B. • The observer is now unable to see runner B.	• Each nerve fiber within the nerve conducts at a slightly different rate. • There is a greater asynchrony in the times when impulses arrive, resulting in mathematical cancellation of potentials that artificially decrease amplitude.	• Where is runner C? (hidden behind runner B) A B C

- **How to account for temporal dispersion and phase cancellation**
  - These normal physiologic concepts are amplified under any pathological condition that prolongs the time needed to reach the recording electrode.
  - **Conduction block** occurs when there is demyelination across a nerve segment, resulting in a greater than 50% loss of the AUC of a CMAP when stimulating at a proximal compared to the distal site.
  - Demyelination and conduction block increase asynchrony between potentials, allowing for greater overlap between negative and positive phases and hence more phase cancellation, even in CMAPs.
  - Therefore, when assessing neuropathies, demonstrating abnormal temporal dispersion, phase cancellation, and conduction block signify a demyelinating lesion.
  - In certain inherited demyelinating neuropathies, such as Charcot Marie tooth type 1, there is uniform slowing of all nerve fibers; therefore, temporal dispersion and conduction block are not prominent features.

- A condition such as acute idiopathic demyelinating neuropathy (AIDP) classically demonstrates features of temporal dispersion and conduction block due to areas of focal demyelination along various nerves.
- When assessing a peripheral nerve injury or entrapment, looking for conduction block or significant temporal dispersion in a proximal compared to a distal site can indicate a demyelinating lesion (and a better prognosis) than a lesion in which both the distal and proximal AUC is reduced (which would signify axonal loss).

Clinical Pearls
- A DEMYELINATING nerve lesion results in increased temporal dispersion, phase cancellation, and conduction block. Prognosis is better because there is limited, if any, axon loss.
- An AXONAL nerve lesion shows reduction in the AUC with both distal as well as proximal stimulation signifying loss of axons. Prognosis is worse due to loss of axons.

QUESTIONS

1. Which nerve stimulation site will exhibit the greatest amount of temporal dispersion?
   A. SNAP of the medial nerve at the wrist
   B. CMAP of the median nerve at the wrist
   C. SNAP of the median nerve at the elbow
   D. CMAP of the median nerve at the elbow

2. Which clinical condition is most likely to have findings of temporal dispersion and phase cancellation?
   A. Amyotrophic lateral sclerosis
   B. Guillain–Barré syndrome
   C. Lambert–Eaton syndrome
   D. Carpal tunnel syndrome

3. What are the classic nerve conduction findings in a patient with chronic inflammatory demyelinating polyradiculoneuropathy?
   A. Uniform conduction velocity slowing
   B. Multifocal conduction block
   C. Pathologic temporal dispersion in multiple motor nerve segments
   D. B and C
   E. All of the above

Answers to the questions are located in Chapter 35.

4. Phase cancellation displays its greatest effect in:
   A. SNAPs due to slight latency differences and variability in conduction speeds compared with CMAPs.
   B. CMAPs due to a longer duration of conduction velocity when compared with SNAPs.
   C. SNAPs spanning over shorter distances.
   D. CMAPs with high AUCs.

5. On routine nerve conduction studies of the ulnar motor nerve, with pickup over the abductor digit minimi, a motor compound muscle action potential (CMAP) at the wrist is 9 mv and below the elbow is 9 mv, whereas *above* the elbow CMAP is 2 mv despite supramaximal stimulation. This most likely signifies:
   A. An axonal lesion at the elbow
   B. A demyelinating lesion at the elbow
   C. A better prognosis
   D. A worse prognosis
   E. A and D are correct
   F. B and C are correct
   G. None are correct

REFERENCES

1. Oh SJ, Kim DE, Kuruoglu HR. What is the best diagnostic index of conduction block and temporal dispersion? *Muscle Nerve*. 1994;17(5):489–493. doi:10.1002/mus.880170504
2. Van Asseldonk JT, Van den Berg LH, Wieneke GH, et al. Criteria for conduction block based on computer simulation studies of nerve conduction with human data obtained in the forearm segment of the median nerve. *Brain*. 2006;129(Pt 9):2447–2460. doi:10.1093/brain/awl197

16

Interpreting Studies

Joelle Gabet and Wendy M. Helkowski

INTRODUCTION
- Nerve conduction and needle examination interpretation require knowledge of normal values and understanding of the significance of variations from normal.
- Abnormalities can help diagnose a focal neuropathy, distinguish a demyelinating neuropathy from an axonal neuropathy, and detect a myopathic process.

NERVE CONDUCTION STUDY INTERPRETATION
Where Is the Lesion?
- Nerve conductions can be used to determine whether the lesion is distal, proximal, or segmental.
- Distal (or onset) latency can be used to determine whether the lesion is **distal**. If the latency measure is *greater than* the normative value for your lab, it is considered prolonged. This is consistent with slowing along the distal segment of the nerve. There are two types of distal latencies that can be calculated:
  - *Distal or onset latency:* The time interval from stimulation to the initial deflection of the waveform (Figure 16.1).
    - Motor nerve conduction studies (NCSs) typically use onset latency for assessment. It is a measure of the fastest conducting motor fibers.
    - Motor NCS is not a "pure" test of time required for the motor nerve to travel because it accounts for the time required for the electrical signal to travel from the stimulus site through the nerve segment *and* the time required to cross the neuromuscular junction (NMJ) *and* the time required for the muscle–cell membranes to depolarize.
  - *Peak latency:* The time interval from stimulation to the peak of the waveform (see Figure 16.1).
    - Sensory NCS typically use peak latency for assessment because the responses are smaller and it can be challenging to define a clear takeoff point for onset latency.
    - There is no involvement of the NMJ or muscle depolarization, thus latency is more of a "pure" test of time required for the sensory nerve to travel.

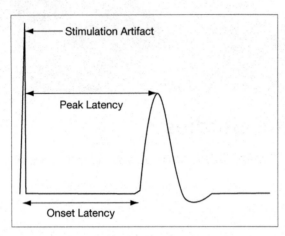

FIGURE 16.1 Latency.

- Conduction velocity can be used to determine whether the lesion is **distal, proximal,** or **segmental**.
  - Velocity is a representation of the speed of the fastest conducting fibers.
    - For motor NCS, two stimulation sites for the same muscle must be used in order to account for the NMJ and muscle depolarization time. The change in distance divided by the change in time can then be calculated.
    - For sensory NCS, this is more directly calculated by dividing the distance traveled by the onset latency. Peak latency cannot be used to calculate conduction velocity.
  - Normal values for conduction velocity:
    - *Upper limbs:* Greater than 50 m/s
    - *Lower limbs:* Greater than 40 m/s
  - If the value for velocity is *less than* the normal value, it is considered abnormal, and represents an abnormality across the segment being tested.
    - Case example: Ulnar neuropathy
    - Compression of the ulnar nerve in the cubital tunnel can be determined by comparing the conduction velocity of the ulnar nerve across the elbow to the distal conduction velocity in the forearm and the proximal conduction velocity in the upper arm. Slowing of more than 12 m/s at the elbow in comparison with the wrist or upper arm is consistent with this segmental compression.

Is Axon Loss or Conduction Block Present?

- Amplitude can be used to determine whether axon loss, conduction block, or both are present along a nerve segment.
- Amplitude is defined as the maximum height of the response, as measured from baseline to peak, or peak to trough (Figure 16.2).

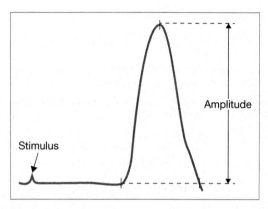

FIGURE 16.2 Amplitude.

- Normal amplitude values vary by lab, and are equal to or greater than the value listed on a table of normal values. Axon loss, conduction block, or both may cause amplitude *less than* the normative values.
  - *Axon loss*—The amplitude will be abnormal with stimulation both proximal and distal to the site of injury, secondary to Wallerian degeneration and death of the entire axon distal to the site of injury.
  - *Conduction block*—The amplitude will be decreased if stimulation occurs proximal to the injury, and normal if stimulation occurs distal to the injury. This is secondary to a focal demyelination severe enough to "block" some or all conduction past that point. A proximal amplitude decrease of 20% or more than the distal amplitude is consistent with conduction block in most motor nerves.
  - *Axon loss with conduction block*—The amplitude with stimulation both proximal and distal to the injury will be decreased due to axon loss. The amplitude with proximal stimulation will be decreased to a greater degree and by at least 20%, due to concomitant conduction block.

What Type of Lesion Is It?

- Nerve conductions can help determine whether the lesion is neuropathic or myopathic.
  - Neuropathic lesions can be located more proximally, such as in radiculopathy, or more distally, such as in plexopathy. In radiculopathy, the sensory NCS is normal, because the dorsal root ganglion is proximal to the injury, resulting in Wallerian degeneration of both sensory and motor axons.
  - In myopathic lesions, the sensory and motor NCS are typically normal, and EMG is needed for diagnosis. However, in distal myopathies or severe myopathies in which both proximal and distal muscles are affected, the motor NCS may have low amplitudes.
- Case examples: Some neuropathies can be defined as primarily motor or primarily sensory.
  - Primarily sensory—Friedrich ataxia: NCS findings typically demonstrate decreased or absent sensory potentials, and normal motor potentials.
  - Primarily motor—Multifocal motor neuropathy: NCS findings typically demonstrate conduction block on motor conduction studies, and normal sensory potentials.

How Long Has the Lesion Been Present?
- After nerve injury, motor axons may remain excitable for up to 7 days, and sensory axons may remain excitable for up to 11 days.
  - With even severe proximal nerve injury, stimulation **distal** to the injury may result in normal or only mildly abnormal values during this time period.
  - Stimulation **proximal** to the site of injury will result in absent responses in both motor and sensory studies, making it difficult to distinguish axonal loss versus conduction block.
- It is thus recommended to wait 10 to 14 days after the injury before performing NCS, as the difference in pathology becomes more clear after this time.

What Are Factors That Limit Interpretation of NCS?
- Decrease in limb temperature could prolong latency, increase amplitude, and decrease conduction velocity.
- Measurement error of distance could limit the calculated conduction velocity.
- Anatomic anomalies may lead to unexpected sensory and motor NCS findings.
- Edema or subcutaneous tissue could impact the level of stimulation, leading to falsely decreased amplitudes.

NEEDLE EMG INTERPRETATION
Components of Needle EMG
There are four components of needle EMG that are used to guide interpretation: insertional activity, motor unit morphology, motor unit recruitment, and pattern of muscle abnormalities.
- **Insertional activity:** The electrical activity associated with movement of the needle through the muscle and for several seconds after stopping needle movement:
  - Normal: A normal electrical signal with movement of the needle in muscle with no prolonged activity after stopping needle movement—except in the neuromuscular end plate region, where miniature end plate potentials and end plate spikes may be seen after needle movement is stopped
    - ☐ Seen in normal muscle, reinnervation, old denervation, myopathy, NMJ disorders
  - Increased: Continued electrical activity after stopping needle movement
    - ☐ Positive waves and fibrillations indicate denervation
    - ☐ Complex repetitive discharges may be seen in chronic denervation
    - ☐ Myotonia associated with myotonia congenita, myotonic dystrophy, and neuropathic disorders (i.e., radiculopathy)
  - Decreased: Lower amplitude and muted sound of electrical activity with needle movement through muscle
    - ☐ Seen in fibrous replacement of muscle tissue in old denervation, chronic myopathy, and rhabdomyolysis

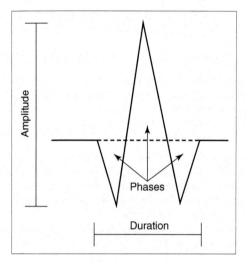

FIGURE 16.3 Motor unit.

- **Motor unit morphology:** Number of phases, duration, and amplitude (Figure 16.3):
  - Phases—Number of baseline crossings plus one
    - Four or less phases is a normal finding
      - Seen in normal muscle, recent denervation (<6 weeks), NMJ
    - Five or more phases are polyphasic and abnormal
      - Seen in nerve sprouting/reinnervation and myopathy
  - Duration (5–15 ms is generally normal, but varies by muscle)
    - Normal in normal muscle, early denervation, and old reinnervation
    - Increased in chronic denervation and associated with polyphasic potentials
    - Decreased in myopathy
  - Amplitude (200–2,000 µV is generally normal, but varies by muscle)
    - Normal in normal muscle, early and chronic denervation with reinnervation
    - Increased in old reinnervation
    - Decreased in myopathy
- **Motor unit recruitment:** Repeated firing of motor units during muscle activation
  - Decreased: Rapid firing frequency of fewer motor units; seen with conduction block or denervation
  - Increased: Early firing of many motor units with minimal force generated; seen with myopathy
  - May be normal in mild denervation or mild myopathy
- **Pattern of muscles involved**

  Focal mononeuropathy
  - **Two or more abnormal muscles** innervated by the **same peripheral nerve but by different nerve roots** (e.g., in a median mononeuropathy, the median-innervated

flexor carpi radialis [C6, C7] and abductor pollicis brevis [C8, T1] are abnormal but the radial-innervated triceps [C6–8] and ulnar-innervated abductor digiti minimi [C8, T1] are normal)

Radiculopathy
- **Two or more abnormal muscles** innervated by the **same nerve root** but innervated by **different peripheral nerves** (e.g., tibialis anterior [L4, L5, deep fibular nerve] and tensor fascia lata [L5, S1, superior gluteal nerve] would both be abnormal in L5 radiculopathy. Muscles without L5 innervation would be normal)

Plexopathy
- Requires a knowledge of the brachial and lumbosacral plexi (e.g., in a posterior cord lesion, the deltoid [C5, C6, upper trunk, posterior cord, axillary nerve] and extensor indicis [C7, C8, middle and lower trunks, posterior cord, radial nerve] would be abnormal; other muscles supplied by the same cervical roots and trunks, but by the medial and lateral cords would be normal)
- Common patterns include abnormal muscles affecting one cord, one trunk, or several isolated nerves from the plexus

Peripheral neuropathy
- More than one **abnormal muscle** innervated by **different peripheral nerves and roots distally**, with **sparing of proximal muscles innervated by the same peripheral nerves and roots** (e.g., the deep fibular-innervated extensor digitorum brevis in the foot is abnormal, but the tibialis anterior which also has deep fibular nerve supply is normal)

Myopathy
- Commonly affects proximal upper and lower limb muscles symmetrically; more distal muscles are typically normal

Needle Exam Changes Over Time After Axonal Nerve Injury

- Immediately
  - **Decreased recruitment of normal-appearing motor units**
  - Normal insertional activity—It takes 1 to 6 weeks after a nerve injury for Wallerian degeneration and muscle membrane instability to occur so there will not be any fibrillations or positive sharp waves yet
- 1 to 3 weeks
  - Decreased recruitment as previously described
  - **Denervation of the paraspinal muscles.** Because the paraspinal muscles are the most proximal muscles, they are the first to show signs of denervation; paraspinal muscles may have positive sharp waves and fibrillations starting 1 to 2 weeks after the acute injury
- 3 to 6 weeks
  - Decreased recruitment and paraspinal muscle denervation as previously described
  - **Active denervation of limb muscles.** At 3 to 6 weeks, Wallerian degeneration has occurred and positive sharp waves and fibrillations appear in the distal muscles; abnormalities will be seen last in the foot and hand muscles
- 6 weeks to 1 year
  - Decreased recruitment as described previously
  - Positive waves and fibrillations disappear as muscle fibers are reinnervated

- **Motor units with long duration and polyphasia.** Six weeks to several months after the injury, axonal sprouting occurs; this means that the remaining axons will now be innervating muscle fibers that were denervated; because the newly formed nerve sprouts innervating these muscle fibers conduct more slowly, they will not fire synchronously with the rest of the muscle fibers innervated by the motor unit; therefore, the motor unit morphology will have longer durations with increased phases

- 1 or more years
  - Decreased recruitment as described previously
  - Polyphasic motor unit becomes triphasic because motor units now have mature myelin on the sprouts that reinnervated denervated muscle fibers and the fibers fire synchronously
  - Motor units have large amplitudes because of the synchronous firing of the larger number of muscle fibers

QUESTIONS

1. What is the minimum amount of time that you should wait after suspected injury before performing nerve conduction studies?
   A. 1 week
   B. 2 weeks
   C. 3 weeks
   D. 4 weeks

2. On evaluation by nerve conduction study (NCS), the amplitude is found to be diminished when measured both proximal and distal to the site of injury. The amplitude with proximal stimulation is also noted to be 10% less than that with distal stimulation. What type of nerve injury does this represent?
   A. Axon loss
   B. Conduction block
   C. Axon loss with conduction block
   D. Peripheral neuropathy

3. A 45-year-old man presents for EMG/nerve conduction study with a history of low-back pain radiating down the left leg to the great toe for the past 2 weeks. What are the expected needle examination findings?
   A. Normal leg and paraspinal muscles
   B. Increased insertional activity with positive waves and fibrillations in the L5-innervated paraspinal muscles
   C. Increased insertional activity with positive waves and fibrillations in the L5-innervated limb muscles
   D. Normal insertional activity with long duration polyphasic potentials in the L5-innervated limb muscles

---

Answers to the questions are located in Chapter 35.

4. A 68-year old woman presents with difficulty climbing stairs and rising from a chair as well as difficulty raising her arms to comb her hair. What needle examination findings in the proximal upper and lower limb muscles would help confirm myopathy as a diagnosis?
   A. Large amplitude polyphasic motor unit potentials with decreased recruitment
   B. Normal findings
   C. Increased insertional activity with positive waves and fibrillations
   D. Small amplitude polyphasic motor unit potentials with increased recruitment

17

Common Anomalies

Nabela Enam and Nigel Shenoy

INTRODUCTION

Anomalous innervations are common, and can lead to unexpected findings on nerve conduction studies (NCS). Recognition is crucial to avoid erroneous interpretation.

- If an anomalous innervation is suspected, look for and rule out technical errors (Table 17.1).
  - Submaximal stimulation, stimulating off the site of the nerve, and poor placement over the muscle belly all may give some NCS findings that are similar to those found with anomalous innervation.

TABLE 17.1 Common Technical Errors

Observation	Possible Error
Increased proximal amplitude	Submaximal stimulation at distal site
Decreased amplitude and/or initial positive (downward) deflection of compound muscle action potential waveform	Suboptimal stimulating electrode placement (i.e., stimulating off the nerve site)
Inconsistently decreased amplitude	Recording electrodes off motor point (i.e., suboptimal electrode placement over muscle belly)
Change in morphology and amplitude	Volume conduction/stimulus spread (i.e., stimulating neighboring nerves or muscles)

- Once technical errors are excluded, common NCS findings that could suggest anomalous innervation include:
  - Lower *compound muscle action potential (CMAP)* amplitude at the distal site compared with the proximal stimulation site
  - Initial positive deflection in CMAP waveform
  - Abnormally low CMAP amplitude with supramaximal stimulation
  - Abnormal waveform morphology for the nerve or muscle being studied

ANATOMY

In the upper limb, the ulnar nerve is derived from the medial cord, whereas the median nerve receives contributions from the medial and lateral cords. The median and ulnar nerves are usually separate, unconnected structures. Figure 17.1 compares the anatomic variation seen in some common upper extremity anomalies.

MARTIN–GRUBER ANASTOMOSIS

Martin–Gruber anastomosis (MGA) is a common anomaly with a prevalence of about 25% (1–4) (see Figure 17.1). It has an autosomal dominant (5) inheritance pattern. Fundamentally, it is C8/T1 ulnar nerve motor fibers that run with the median nerve proximally until they finally cross back over to the ulnar nerve in the forearm. This is called a *median-to-ulnar crossover*. Ninety-one percent of cases supply the anterior interosseous nerve (6) and 68% of cases are bilateral (7) (Table 17.2).

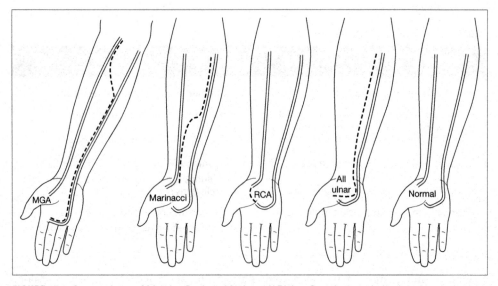

FIGURE 17.1 Comparison of Martin–Gruber, Marinacci, Riche–Cannieu, and all-ulnar hand anomalies, all represented by dashed lines in the upper limb.

MGA, Martin–Gruber anastomosis; RCA, Riche–Cannieu anomaly.

TABLE 17.2 Nerve Conduction Study Findings in Martin–Gruber Anastomosis

Site Stimulated/Pickup	Nerve Fibers Contributing	Waveform Comparison
A. Median elbow/APB	Median + MGA	
B. Median wrist/APB	Median	
C. Median elbow/FDI	MGA	
D. Ulnar elbow/FDI	Ulnar	
E. Median wrist/FDI	None	
F. Ulnar wrist/FDI	Ulnar + MGA	

APB, abductor pollicis brevis; FDI, first dorsal interosseous; MGA, Martin–Gruber anastomosis.

Note: Waveform variation between median and ulnar nerve stimulation at elbow and wrist sites in the presence of MGA. A and B represent pickup over the APB, with A demonstrating an increased proximal amplitude because it contains both MGA and median fibers, whereas B only contains median fibers. C to F represent pickup over the FDI muscle. C demonstrates stimulating the median nerve at the elbow and carrying only the MGA fibers. D shows ulnar nerve stimulation at the elbow and contains only ulnar nerve fibers. E demonstrates stimulation of the median nerve at the wrist site. F represents stimulation of the ulnar nerve at the wrist, containing both ulnar and MGA fibers.

- MGA occurs as a combination of three types:
  - *Type I:* MGA fibers supply the hypothenar muscles in 41% to 61% of cases (1)
  - *Type II:* Fibers end at FDI in 95% to 100% of cases (1)
  - *Type III:* Fibers supply the adductor pollicis (AP) and deep head of the flexor pollicis brevis (FPB) in 14% of cases (1)

Electrodiagnostic Findings in Martin–Gruber Anastomosis

- Often the initial finding in MGA will be a positive deflection, or a larger amplitude, of the CMAP when studying the median nerve at the elbow with pickup at the abductor pollicis brevis (APB). MGA does not innervate the APB; however, it does innervate the AP and the deep head of the FPB, which are also located at the thenar eminence and alter the CMAP recording over the APB (larger amplitude or initial positive deflection) (Table 17.3).

When to Think About MGA

TABLE 17.3 Nerve Conduction Study Clues to Suggest Martin–Gruber Anastomosis

Electrodiagnostic Finding	Comment
Decreased ulnar CMAP at elbow stimulation compared with wrist	May mimic ulnar conduction block (sometimes referred to as *pseudo-conduction block*)
Increased median CMAP at elbow compared with wrist stimulation	Ensure that median wrist stimulation is supramaximal
Initial positive deflection of median CMAP waveform	Ensure that recording electrodes are on the motor point of abductor pollicis brevis
Abnormally fast conduction velocity across forearm segment of median nerve in patients with CTS	Confirm CTS with sensory and comparison studies

CMAP, compound muscle action potential; CTS, carpal tunnel syndrome.

- Confirmatory studies:
  - Stimulate median and ulnar wrist and elbow while recording electrodes over FDI.
  - A CMAP response from median stimulation at the elbow (wrist/FDI pickup) will be present if MGA is present.
  - Ulnar wrist CMAP amplitude (ulnar and MGA fibers) will be significantly higher than ulnar elbow CMAP amplitude (ulnar fibers only), and may be perceived as conduction block. It is, however, a pseudoconduction block because the ulnar elbow stimulation activates only ulnar fibers, whereas the ulnar wrist stimulation activates ulnar and MGA nerve fibers.
  - Median stimulation at elbow with pickup over FDI contains only the MGA nerve fiber contribution.
  - A second channel can be used while stimulating at the median elbow to observe coactivation in the hypothenar or other muscle groups.
- Clinical significance:
  - In patients with an ulnar neuropathy proximal to MGA crossover, intrinsic hand weakness will be less severe. A median nerve lesion proximal to crossover in the elbow could lead to some intrinsic hand weakness.

MARINACCI ANOMALY

A similar communication to the MGA in the upper extremity is the Marinacci anastomosis, which occurs when there is an ulnar to median crossover in the distal forearm. This is less common than an MGA with a reported prevalence of 4% (see Figure 17.1) (8).

RICHE–CANNIEU ANOMALY

The deep branch of the ulnar nerve in the hand crosses over to the recurrent median nerve in the hand (see Figure 17.1). This results in dual innervation of thenar muscles or predominantly ulnar innervation of thenar muscles. It is common and may occur in up to 80% of hands (9). Due to the dual innervation of the thenar musculature, it may not be immediately obvious on routine NCS (Table 17.4).

TABLE 17.4 Nerve Conduction Study Findings in Riche–Cannieu Anomaly With Concomitant CTS

Site Stimulated/Pickup	Nerve Fibers Contributing	Waveform Comparison
A—Median elbow/APB	Median reduced from CTS	A
B—Median wrist/APB	Median reduced from CTS	B
C—Ulnar elbow/APB	RCA	C
D—Ulnar wrist/APB	RCA	D

ABP, abductor pollicis brevis; CTS, carpal tunnel syndrome; RCA, Riche–Cannieu anomaly.

Note: Waveform variation between median and ulnar nerve stimulation at elbow and wrist sites in the presence of the RCA and CTS. A to D represent pickup over the APB muscle. Stimulating the median nerve at either the elbow (A) or the wrist (B) delivers a smaller than anticipated amplitude in the presence of CTS. Stimulation of the ulnar nerve at the elbow (C) or the wrist (D) demonstrates a larger amplitude, as the ulnar nerve is delivering portions of the signal to the thenar eminence via the RCA without being affected by CTS.

Electrodiagnostic Findings in Riche–Cannieu Anomaly

- Confirmatory studies (Table 17.5):
  - After performing routine ulnar and median motor NCS, keep the surface recording electrodes on APB while stimulating the ulnar nerve at the wrist and elbow, taking care to avoid volume conduction to the median nerve. If Riche–Cannieu anomaly is present, a CMAP will be present recording over the APB with ulnar wrist and elbow stimulation.
  - The CMAP at APB can also be recorded with needle electrode, stimulating the ulnar and median nerves.
  - An additional channel can be used to confirm that a single ulnar stimulation causes a hypothenar CMAP (with surface recording) and APB CMAP with needle recording.
- Clinical significance of Riche–Cannieu anomaly:
  - Severe median nerve lesions, especially at the wrist, can spare the thenar muscles.
  - Ulnar neuropathy can present as a C8–T1 lesion on needle EMG due to denervation potentials in both ulnar intrinsic and thenar muscles (10).

TABLE 17.5 Electrodiagnostic Clues to Suggest Riche–Cannieu Anomaly

Electrodiagnostic Finding	Comment
Low CMAP at APB with median nerve wrist and elbow stimulation	Ensure that median wrist stimulation is supramaximal.
Occasionally the waveform of the median CMAP will have increased duration and a biphasic appearance	Ensure that recording electrodes are on the motor point of APB.
EMG denervation potentials in APB in the clinical setting of ulnar neuropathy	Ensure that needle electrode is not in an ulnar-innervated thenar muscle. Rule out other causes like C8–T1 radiculopathy or concomitant median neuropathy.
APB, abductor pollicis brevis; CMAP, compound muscle action potential.	

ALL-ULNAR HAND

The all-ulnar hand is a rare finding, in which the thenar and other intrinsic hand muscles are all innervated only by the ulnar nerve. This is an ulnar-to-median anastomosis. On NCS there may be little or no evoked motor response with stimulation of the median nerve, but a decent CMAP is seen with ulnar stimulation picking up over the APB. This is a rare anomaly and it is important to avoid volume conduction with any wrist stimulation (see Figure 17.1).

ACCESSORY FIBULAR NERVE

The AFN is a branch of the superficial fibular nerve that splits at the fibular head toward the lateral malleolus and innervates the extensor digitorum brevis (EDB). This results in dual innervation of the EDB from deep and AFN. It has an autosomal dominant inheritance pattern (11), prevalence of about 28%, and is bilateral in 57% of cases (Table 17.6) (12).

When to Think About Accessory Fibular Nerve

TABLE 17.6 Electrodiagnostic Clues to Suggest Accessory Fibular Nerve

Electrodiagnostic or Exam Finding	Comment
Larger CMAPs are seen at fibular head and popliteal fossa compared to ankle stimulation of fibular nerve.	• Ensure that ankle fibular nerve stimulation is supramaximal. • Popliteal stimulus is not volume conducted to tibial nerve, which can cause change in CMAP morphology and falsely elevated proximal fibular CMAP amplitude.
Patient has clinical footdrop with tibialis anterior weakness, but preserved extensor digitorum brevis activation.	• Ensure that fibularis longus and brevis are normal.
CMAP, compound muscle action potential.	

Electrodiagnostic Findings in Accessory Fibular Nerve

- Confirmatory studies (Table 17.7):
  - Perform basic fibular and tibial NCS. If there is an increased amplitude at fibular head stimulation, stimulate the AFN at the lateral malleolus, recording over the EDB.
  - If AFN is present, there will be a response generated from stimulation at the lateral malleolus. The deep fibular nerve ankle stimulation plus the AFN simulation will be mildly higher than stimulation at the fibular head.
  - Avoid overstimulation at the lateral malleolus to prevent volume conduction.
- Clinical significance of AFN:
  - Deep fibular nerve lesions may appear incomplete due to dual innervation of EDB by the deep and AFNs.

TABLE 17.7 Nerve Conduction Study Findings With Accessory Fibular Nerve

Site Stimulated/Pickup	Nerve Fibers Contributing	Waveform Comparison
A. Fibular head/EDB	Deep fibular + AFN	
B. Anterior ankle/EDB	Deep fibular	
C. Lateral malleolus/EDB	AFN	

AFN, accessory fibular nerve; EDB, extensor digitorum brevis.

Waveform variation seen with stimulation of fibular nerve at fibular head, anterior ankle, and lateral malleolus in the presence of an AFN. A to C represent pickup over the EDB. Stimulating at the fibular head (A) will have maximal amplitude because it contains fibers that travel through both the deep fibular and the AFN. The amplitude of A will equal the summation of stimulating the deep fibular nerve at the ankle (B) and the AFN posterior to the lateral malleolus (C). An AFN should always be considered whenever proximal stimulation of the fibular nerve (A) has a larger amplitude than the distal stimulation (B), thus prompting stimulation behind the lateral malleolus.

QUESTIONS

1. In the presence of a Martin–Gruber anastomosis (MGA), which of the following stimulation sites, recording at the first dorsal interosseous (FDI), has contribution to its compound motor action potential (CMAP) amplitude from MGA fibers?
   A. Median wrist stimulation
   B. Ulnar wrist stimulation
   C. Ulnar elbow stimulation
   D. Both A and C

2. A patient with documented ulnar neuropathy at the left elbow has a better prognosis for motor preservation in the intrinsic hand muscles with which of the following conditions?
   A. MGA in the forearm segment
   B. An ulnar to median crossover in the forearm
   C. Riche–Cannieu anomaly in the left hand
   D. Both A and C

Answers to the questions are located in Chapter 35.

3. A 26-year-old female patient has denervation potentials on EMG of the abductor digiti minimi (ADM), abductor pollicis brevis (APB), and first dorsal interosseous (FDI), as well as normal cervical paraspinal EMG findings. What additional electrodiagnostic study would help differentiate between a brachial plexopathy and an anomalous innervation?
   A. Medial antebrachial cutaneous nerve conduction study
   B. Needle recording of ADM CMAP while stimulating the median nerve at the wrist
   C. Needle recording of APB CMAP while stimulating the ulnar nerve at the wrist
   D. Both A and C

4. A patient has a suspected accessory fibular nerve. Which of the follow actions on nerve conduction studies will further elucidate the diagnosis?
   A. Confirm that the ankle stimulation is supramaximal
   B. Increase pulse width to ensure that the popliteal stimulation is supramaximal
   C. Stimulate at the medial malleolus
   D. Both A and C

REFERENCES

1. Gutmann L. Median-ulnar nerve communication and carpal tunnel syndrome. *J Neurol Neurosurg Psychiatry*. 1970;40:982–986. PubMed PMID: 201732.
2. Erdem HR, Ergun S, Erturk C, et al. Electrophysiological evaluation of the incidence of Martin-Gruber anastomosis in healthy subjects. *Yonsei Med J*. 2002;43(3):291–295. doi:10.3349/ymj.2002.43.3.291
3. Hasegawa O, Matsumoto S, Iino M, et al. Prevalence of Martin-Gruber anastomosis on motor nerve conduction studies [in Japanese]. *No To Shinkei*. 2001;53(2):161–164. PubMed PMID: 11268580.
4. Taams KO. Martin–Gruber connections in South Africa. An anatomical study. *J Hand Surg Br*. 1997;22(3):328–330. PubMed PMID: 9222911.
5. Crutchfield CA, Gutmann L. Hereditary aspects of median-ulnar nerve communications. *J Neurol Neurosurg Psychiatry*. 1980;43:53–55. PubMed PMID: 7354357.
6. Srinivasan R, Rhodes J. The median ulnar anastomosis (Martin Gruber) in normal and congenitally abnormal fetuses. *Arch Neurol*. 1981;38:418–419. PubMed PMID: 6454405.
7. Kimura J, Murphy MJ, Varda DJ. Electrophysiological study of anomalous innervation of intrinsic hand muscles. *Arch Neurol*. 1976;33:842–844. PubMed PMID: 999546.
8. Koo YS, Cho C, Kim BJ. Pitfalls in using electrophysiological studies to diagnose neuromuscular disorders. *J Clin Neurol*. 2012;8:1–14. doi:10.3988/jcn.2012.8.1.1
9. Kimura I, Ayyar DR, Lippmann SM. Electrophysiological verification of the ulnar to median nerve communications in the hand and forearm. *Tohoku J Exp Med*. 1983;141(3):269–274. PubMed PMID: 6316583.
10. Dumitru D, Walsh NE, Weber CF. Electrophysiologic study of Riche Cannieu anomaly. *Electromyogr Clin Neurophysiol*. 1988;28:27–31. PubMed PMID: 3168913.
11. Crutchfield CA, Gutmann L. Hereditary aspects of accessory deep peroneal nerve. *J Neurol Neurosurg Psychiatry*. 1973;36:989–990. PubMed PMID: 4772729.
12. Neundorfer B, Seiberth R. The accessory deep peroneal nerve. *J Neurol*. 1975;209:125–129. PubMed PMID: 51049.

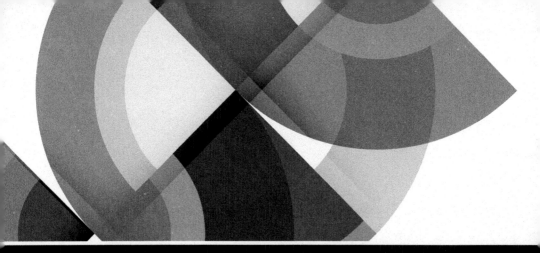

V COMMON CLINICAL ENTITIES

18

Carpal Tunnel Syndrome

Leslie Rydberg

INTRODUCTION

Median mononeuropathy at the wrist is the electrodiagnostic (EDX) equivalent to carpal tunnel syndrome (CTS), which is a clinical entity. It is the most common peripheral entrapment neuropathy. Epidemiological studies reveal an incidence between 1.5 and 3.5 per 1,000 person-years (1). Therefore, it is not surprising that one of the most common reasons for referral to an EDX laboratory is for evaluation for possible CTS.

CLINICAL PRESENTATION

Although most cases of CTS are idiopathic (often related to occupation or repetitive stress), compression of the median nerve at the wrist can also arise from:

- Space-occupying lesions: Arthritis, fracture, ganglion cyst
- Increased volume in the carpal tunnel: Pregnancy; thyroid, cardiac, or renal disease
- Double crush syndrome: Coexistent cervical radiculopathy and CTS

    Regardless of the cause, compression of the median nerve in the carpal tunnel has a characteristic progression. Key elements in the history:
    - Paresthesias
    - Pain, often at night
    - Thumb/hand weakness
    - Decline in function
    - "Flick" sign, patient reports shaking or flicking the hand(s), often at night
- Key findings on physical examination:
    - Sensory: Decreased sensation of the lateral 3½ digits with splitting of the 4th digit
    - Motor: Weakness of thumb abduction or opposition, atrophy of the thenar eminence
    - Provocative tests:
        - Phalen's—Hold the wrist at 90° of flexion for 30 to 60 seconds
        - Tinel's—Tap over the median nerve in the carpal tunnel

ANATOMY OF THE CARPAL TUNNEL

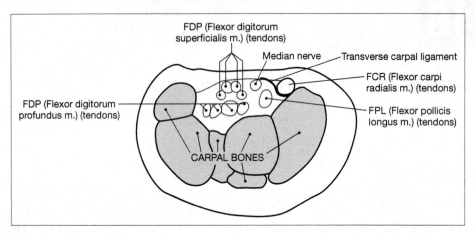

FIGURE 18.1 Anatomy of the carpal tunnel.
Source: From Cuccurullo SJ. *Physical Medicine and Rehabilitation Board Review.* 2nd ed. New York, NY: Demos Medical Publishing; 2010:401.

- Floor and sides: Carpal bones
- Roof: Transverse carpal ligament
- Contents:
  - Median nerve, tendons of flexor pollicis longus (FPL), flexor digitorum superficialis (FDS), and flexor digitorum profundus (FDP) muscles

Motor Portion

After the median nerve passes through the carpal tunnel, the motor portion splits into the recurrent and the direct branches.

- Recurrent branch: Opponens pollicis, abductor pollicis brevis (APB), and superficial head of the flexor pollicis brevis
- Direct branch: The two lateral lumbricals

Sensory Portion

The median nerves give off the palmar cutaneous branch before entering the carpal tunnel, so only the palmar digital sensory branch travels through the tunnel.

ELECTRODIAGNOSTIC APPROACH

EDX testing enables the clinician to determine the functional status of the sensory and motor components of the median nerve at the wrist (2).

- Nerve conduction studies:
  - Identify focal slowing or conduction block in the carpal tunnel
  - Exclude the presence of a more proximal median neuropathy, polyneuropathy, or brachial plexopathy
- Electromyography:
  - Determine whether there is axonal loss of the median-innervated hand muscles
  - Confirm or deny the presence of a cervical radiculopathy
- Routine nerve conduction studies:
  - Median motor to APB—Stimulating at the wrist and antecubital fossa
  - Ulnar motor to abductor digiti minimi—Stimulating at the wrist, below elbow, and above elbow
  - Median sensory to digits II or III
  - Ulnar sensory to digit V
- Evidence suggestive of CTS includes prolongation of the distal median sensory and motor latencies and/or reduction in compound muscle action potential (CMAP) or sensory nerve action potential (SNAP) amplitudes.
- Comparison studies (Table 18.1):
  - Used when the clinical suspicion of CTS is high, but the routine nerve conduction studies (NCS) fail to reveal evidence of a median mononeuropathy at the wrist.
  - This is commonly done to compare the latencies of sensory nerves that travel through the carpal tunnel (i.e., median) to sensory nerves that do not travel through the carpal tunnel (i.e., ulnar).
  - A possible supplementary NCS can be done with motor nerve comparisons (i.e., median-innervated second lumbrical compared to ulnar-innervated second interossei).
  - The Combined Sensory Index (CSI), or Robinson Index, combines the values from three comparison studies, which results in increased sensitivity and preserved specificity when compared with each individual test (Table 18.1). Therefore, when combining the differences of the three tests, a smaller total (0.9 ms) can be used than if each of the tests were used individually (1.2 ms).

TABLE 18.1 Combined Sensory Index/Robinson Index

Transcarpal 8 Test *Stimulation* • *Median*—Palm (8 cm distally along a line between the median nerve at the wrist and digits II and III) • *Ulnar*—Palm (8 cm distally along a line between the ulnar nerve at the wrist and digits IV and V) • Recording: Bar electrode placed at the median and ulnar nerves at the wrist, respectively *Significant Difference (ms)* • >0.3	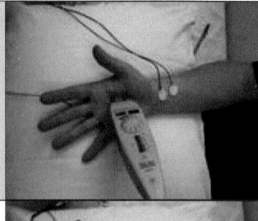
Median Versus Ulnar to Digit IV Test *Stimulation* • *Median*—Wrist (14 cm proximally along the course of the median nerve) • *Ulnar*—Wrist (14 cm proximally along the course of the ulnar nerve) • Recording: Ring electrodes placed on digit IV *Significant Difference (ms)* • >0.4	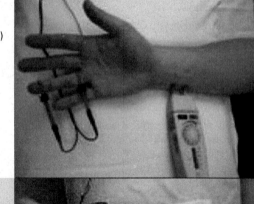
Bactrian (Median Versus Radial to Digit I) Test *Stimulation* • *Median*—Wrist (10 cm proximally along the course of the median nerve) • *Ulnar*—Wrist (10 cm proximally along the course of the radial nerve) • Recording: Ring electrodes placed on digit I *Significant Difference (ms)* • >0.5 **Combined Sensory Index** *Significant Difference (ms)* • Add up the latency differences from all three tests • >0.9	

Source: Robinson LR, Micklesen PJ, Wang L. Strategies for analyzing nerve conduction data: superiority of a summary index over single tests. *Muscle Nerve.* 1998;21:1166–1171. PubMed PMID: 9703442.

Electromyography
- There is no standard algorithm for electromyography testing in the evaluation of CTS.
- The purpose of including the needle study in the evaluation is to rule out a cervical radiculopathy, brachial plexopathy, or proximal median neuropathy, and to determine the extent of axonal involvement in median-innervated muscles.

ASSESSING THE SEVERITY OF CARPAL TUNNEL SYNDROME
- The median sensory nerves are affected earlier in the process and the motor nerves are affected later in the process. In a more severe median mononeuropathy, both sensory and motor NCS are abnormal.
- Myelin function is affected earlier in the process and axons are affected later in the process. In a more severe median mononeuropathy, axonal involvement is seen on NCS and electromyography.
- The correlation between nerve conduction slowing and clinical symptoms in CTS is limited (3). Consequently, the use of EDX findings to comment on the severity of the disease process is controversial. Some feel that the EDX consultant should comment only on the presence of a median mononeuropathy, location of the lesion, presence of demyelination, and/or axonal loss, and if there are any changes from previous studies (4). However, others argue that the degree of nerve injury and the EDX consultant's opinion of the severity of the disease should be included in the report. Finally, some endorse the use of severity scales for research, but not clinical situations. One example of a severity grading scale is the Stevens criteria (Table 18.2).

TABLE 18.2 Stevens Criteria to Assess Carpal Tunnel Syndrome

Mild CTS	Prolonged sensory or mixed nerve distal latency ± decreased SNAP amplitude
Moderate CTS	Abnormal median sensory latencies as listed and prolonged median motor distal latency
Severe CTS	Prolonged motor and sensory distal latencies with any of the following:
	Absent median SNAP
	Low-amplitude or absent median CMAP
	Evidence of abnormal spontaneous activity, reduced recruitment, and motor unit potential changes on needle examination

CMAP, compound muscle action potential; CTS, carpal tunnel syndrome; SNAP, sensory nerve action potential.

Source: Stevens JC. AAEM minimonograph #26: the electrodiagnosis of carpal tunnel syndrome. *Muscle Nerve.* 1997;20:1477–1486. PubMed PMID: 9390659.

QUESTIONS

1. A branch of the median nerve innervates which of the following muscles?
   A. Adductor pollicis
   B. Opponens pollicis
   C. Flexor digitorum profundus to the 4th digit
   D. Extensor pollicis brevis

2. You are performing nerve conduction studies (NCS) on a patient with possible carpal tunnel syndrome (CTS), and you perform the three studies used in the Combined Sensory Index (CSI). Based on the NCS in the table provided, you are able to conclude the following:

Test	Nerve	Distance (cm)	Peak Latency (ms)	Amplitude (µV)
Transcarpal 8 (mixed motor/sensory)	Median	8	2.8	21
	Ulnar	8	2.2	18
Median versus ulnar to digit IV (sensory)	Median	14	3.1	22
	Ulnar	14	2.8	18
Bactrian median versus radial to digit I (sensory)	Median	10	3.4	19
	Radial	10	3.0	16

   A. None of the tests suggest CTS.
   B. All of the tests suggest CTS.
   C. The transcarpal 8 is the only test that suggests CTS.
   D. The transcarpal 8 and the CSI suggest the diagnosis of CTS.

3. A 50-year-old woman presents with numbness and tingling in digits 1 to 3 and thenar atrophy. What do you expect her electrodiagnostic testing to look like?
   A. Absent median sensory nerve action potential with prolonged median motor action potential latency with low amplitude
   B. Normal distal latency in the median sensory nerve action potential with prolonged median motor action potential latency
   C. Prolonged distal latency in the median sensory nerve action potential with normal median motor action potential latency with reduced conduction velocity through the forearm
   D. Prolonged distal latency in the median sensory nerve action potential with normal median motor action potential latency and normal amplitude

---

Answers to the questions are located in Chapter 35.

4. A 60-year-old woman presents with numbness and tingling in digits 1 to 3 and median hand weakness. Why should you perform electromyography in this patient?
   A. To rule out radiculopathy
   B. To assess for axonal injury in the median-innervated muscles
   C. To rule out proximal median neuropathy
   D. All of the above

REFERENCES
1. Wolf JM, Mountcastle S, Owens BD. Incidence of carpal tunnel syndrome in the US military population. *Hand (N Y)*. 2009;4(3):289–293. doi:10.1007/s11552-009-9166-y
2. American Association of Electrodiagnostic Medicine; American Academy of Neurology; American Academy of Physical Medicine and Rehabilitation. Practice parameter for electrodiagnostic studies in carpal tunnel syndrome (summary statement). *Muscle Nerve*. 2002;25:918–922. doi: 10.1002/mus.10185
3. Chan L, Turner JA, Comstock BA, et al. The relationship between electrodiagnostic findings and patient symptoms and function in carpal tunnel syndrome. *Arch Phys Med Rehabil*. 2007;88:19–24. doi:10.1016/j.apmr.2006.10.013
4. Robinson LR, Kliot M. Stop using arbitrary grading schemes in carpal tunnel syndrome. *Muscle Nerve*. 2008;37:804. doi:10.1002/mus.21012

19

Ulnar Neuropathy at the Elbow

Akinpelumi Beckley and Susie S. Kwon

INTRODUCTION

Ulnar neuropathy may result from nerve compression as it traverses along the medial aspect of the arm, crosses the elbow, moves through the forearm, or passes through the wrist as seen in Figure 19.1.

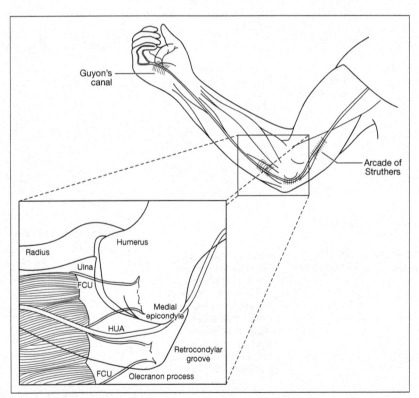

FIGURE 19.1 Ulnar nerve with areas of entrapment.

FCU, flexor carpi ulnaris; HUA, humeroulnar aponeurotic arcade.

CLINICAL PRESENTATION

- Paresthesias in the 4th and 5th digit of the hand
- Weakness of the intrinsic muscles of the hand can be seen leading to syndromes in Table 19.1:

TABLE 19.1 Ulnar Nerve Syndromes

Syndrome	Weak Muscle	Description	
Froment sign	Adductor pollicis	Inability to hold a piece of paper between the thumb and index finger by adducting thumb. Instead, median innervated flexor pollicis longus is substituted with thumb interphalangeal flexion.	**FIGURE 19.2** Froment sign.
Ulnar claw hand	3rd and 4th lumbricals	Hyperextension of the metacarpophalangeal joints and flexion of the proximal interphalangeal and distal interphalangeal joints of digits 4 and 5. This occurs due to unopposed pull from radial innervated extensor digitorum communis.	**FIGURE 19.3** Ulnar claw hand.
Wartenberg sign	Palmar interossei (3rd)	Inability to adduct 5th digit thus finger remains slightly abducted. Unopposed activity of radial innervated extensor digiti minimi. *Differs from Wartenberg syndrome—superficial radial nerve palsy.*	**FIGURE 19.4** Wartenberg sign.

ANATOMY

Ulnar nerve anatomy is summarized in Table 19.2.

- The ulnar nerve is the terminal extension of the medial cord of the brachial plexus, which is derived from the C8 and T1 nerve roots.
- Above the elbow, the ulnar nerve passes through the arcade of Struthers. The nerve then enters the retrocondylar (ulnar) groove adjacent to the medial epicondyle of the elbow, proceeds into the humeroulnar aponeurotic arcade (cubital tunnel). It traverses the forearm prior to entering the wrist via Guyon's canal.
- In the proximal forearm, the nerve gives rise to muscular branches to the flexor carpi ulnaris (FCU) and the medial division to digits 4 and 5 of the flexor digitorum profundus (FDP) (4,5).
- Proximal to the wrist, dorsal and palmer cutaneous nerves branch off of the main nerve.
- When the nerve crosses the wrist at Guyon's canal, superficial digital sensory branches are separate to supply digit 5 and the medial half of digit 4. The deep branch carries motor fibers supplying most of the intrinsic muscles of the hands.

TABLE 19.2 Ulnar Nerve Anatomy

Forearm	Motor		• Flexor carpi ulnaris • Medial half of flexor digitorum profundus
Hand	Motor		
		• Hypothenar	*Palmaris brevis* • Abductor digiti minimi • Opponens digiti minimi • Flexor digiti minimi
		• Thenar	• Adductor pollicis • Deep head of the flexor pollicis brevis
		• Other intrinsics	• Palmar interossei • Dorsal interossei • Medial half of lumbricals
Hand	Sensory		• Palmar ulnar cutaneous (before Guyon's canal) • Dorsal ulnar cutaneous (before Guyon's canal) • Digital branches (after Guyon's canal)

> **Clinical Pearl**
> - Dually innervated muscles in the upper extremity include: FPB, lumbricals, FDP.

ELECTRODIAGNOSTIC APPROACH

Nerve conduction studies (NCS) used to examine motor and sensory nerves in the upper limbs are described in Chapters 4 and 5. Sensory abnormalities along the distribution are helpful in identifying the location of injury as outlined in Table 19.3. Motor conduction studies are especially useful in identifying pathology at the elbow, which is the most common area of injury. The specific techniques for conduction studies of the ulnar nerve are described in Table 19.4. Electrodiagnostic workup for ulnar neuropathy at the elbow is outlined in Table 19.5 and requires careful attention to elbow positioning during measurement and stimulation. When the elbow is extended, the nerve is slack and any measurements taken in this position can result in false slowing. Therefore, when performing ulnar NCS:

- The arm should be abducted to 90° and the elbow flexed to 70° to 90° to obtain the most accurate distance for the ulnar nerve (1).
- Below the elbow, stimulation should be at least 3 cm below the medial epicondyle to include the humeroulnar aponeurotic arcade (cubital tunnel).
- Above the elbow, stimulation should be at least 10 cm proximal from the stimulation site below the elbow.
- Inching is performed by stimulating the nerve every 1 to 2 cm as it traverses from the humeroulnar arcade to the arcade of Struthers to identify an area of focal nerve pathology. Inching is performed if there is a difference in conduction velocity or amplitude across the elbow (2).

TABLE 19.3 Sensory Distributions to Help Distinguish Level of Injury

Peripheral Nerve	Sensory Distribution	May Be Abnormal in the Following
Ulnar digital branches	• Digit 5 and medial half of digit 4	• Ulnar neuropathy at the wrist • Ulnar neuropathy at the elbow • Plexopathy
DUC and PUC	• DUC—Dorsal aspect of the medial hand and dorsum of the medial 1½ digits • PUC—Medial aspect of palm	• Ulnar neuropathy at the elbow • Plexopathy
Medial antebrachial cutaneous	• Volar surface of the medial forearm	• Plexopathy
DUC, dorsal ulnar cutaneous; PUC, palmar ulnar cutaneous.		

TABLE 19.4 Ulnar Study-Specific Nerve Conduction Studies

Test	Setup
Dorsal ulnar cutaneous	• Stimulation site 　▪ Slightly proximal and volar to the ulnar styloid (distance 8–10 cm) with the hand pronated • Recording site 　▪ E1: Over the web space between the 4th and 5th digits 　▪ E2: 3–4 cm distally over the 5th digit
Medial antebrachial cutaneous	• Stimulation site 　▪ Midway between the biceps tendon and the medial epicondyle • Recording site 　▪ E1: 12 cm distal to the stimulation site in line to the ulnar wrist 　▪ E2: 3–4 cm distal to E1
Inching technique	• Stimulation sites 　▪ Stimulate at 2-cm intervals along the ulnar groove • Recording site 　▪ Same as for ulnar motor to the abductor digiti minimi

The landmarks for needle electromyography for the most frequently tested muscles in the workup for ulnar neuropathy are listed in Table 19.6. The findings seen on nerve conduction studies to differentiate axonal and demyelinating lesions are shown in Table 19.7 (1).

TABLE 19.5 Suggested Initial Electrodiagnostic Workup for Ulnar Neuropathy at the Elbow

Nerve Conduction Studies	Needle Electromyography
Motor • Median motor to the APB • Ulnar motor to the ADM, including across the elbow • Consider inching technique across the elbow	Routine ulnar muscles • First dorsal interosseous or ADM • Flexor digitorum profundus or flexor carpi ulnaris
Sensory • Median sensory to digit 2 or 3 • Ulnar sensory to digit 5 • Consider dorsal ulnar cutaneous • Consider medial antebrachial cutaneous	If ulnar muscles are abnormal • At least two non-ulnar lower trunk/C7–C8–T1 muscles: 　▪ APB 　▪ Flexor pollicis longus 　▪ Extensor indicis proprius • C8–T1 paraspinals
Late responses • Median F-response • Ulnar F-response	
ADM, abductor digiti minimi; APB, abductor pollicis brevis.	

TABLE 19.6 Electromyography Landmarks for Frequently Tested Muscles in Ulnar Neuropathy

	Electromyography Landmark	Muscle Activation
C8–T1 Ulnar-Innervated Muscles		
First dorsal interosseous	Dorsal hand, halfway between the first and second MCP joints	Abduct index finger
Abductor digiti minimi	Medial hand, midpoint of 5th MCP	Abduct 5th digit
Flexor carpi ulnaris (also C7)	Medial forearm at the midpoint between elbow and wrist (forearm supinated)	Flex wrist in ulnar deviation or abduct 5th digit
Flexor digitorum profundus 4,5	Three to four fingerbreadths distal to olecranon, superficial (elbow flexed)	Flex distal interphalangeal
C8–T1 Median Innervated Muscle		
Abductor pollicis brevis	Thenar eminence, just lateral to midpoint of first metacarpal	Abduct thumb (arm supinated)
C7–C8 Radial Innervated Muscle		
Extensor indicis proprius	Two fingerbreadths proximal to ulnar styloid (arm pronated)	Extend index finger

MCP, metacarpophalangeal.

TABLE 19.7 Abnormal Nerve Conduction Study Findings in Ulnar Neuropathy at the Elbow May Represent Demyelinating or Axonal Injury

Demyelinating Injury
- *Focal slowing across elbow*
  - Nerve conduction velocity less than 50 m/s between above-elbow and below-elbow stimulation
  - >10 m/s slowing compared to forearm segment
- *Conduction block*
  - Decreased CMAP amplitude or area by 20% when comparing above-elbow with below-elbow stimulation

Axonal Injury
- *Abnormal ulnar digit 5 SNAP*
- *Abnormal dorsal ulnar cutaneous SNAP*
- *Abnormal ulnar CMAP*

CMAP, compound muscle action potential; SNAP, sensory nerve action potential.

QUESTIONS

1. A 40-year-old female complains of numbness and tingling in the 4th and 5th digits after taking up competitive cycling several months ago. She denies any sensory complaints and has no weakness. The lesion is most likely located in:
   A. Medial aspect of the arm
   B. Distal aspect of the humeroulnar arcade
   C. Medial aspect of mid forearm
   D. Guyon's canal

2. A 72-year-old male patient presents to the office complaining of difficulty with buttoning his shirts. You observe that he has difficulty holding a piece of paper between his thumb and index finger and diagnose recognizing a positive Froment sign. This is due to:
   A. Hyperextension of the metacarpophalangeal joints
   B. Substitution of the flexor pollicis longus
   C. Unopposed action of radial innervated extensor digitorum communis
   D. Weakness of the interossei due to compression of the palmar cutaneous nerve

3. A 60-year-old male finds that he is unable to straighten his fingers completely on his right hand. If the lesion is due to ulnar neuropathy in the arcade of Struthers, which of the following muscles would be normal on needle electromyography?
   A. Flexor digitorum profundus
   B. Flexor digiti minimi
   C. Flexor pollicis longus
   D. First dorsal interossei

4. Which of the following nerve injuries would most likely cause a decreased amplitude and conduction velocity in the medial antebrachial cutaneous nerve of the forearm?
   A. Middle trunk of brachial plexus
   B. Medial cord of brachial plexus
   C. Ulnar neuropathy above the elbow at the arcade of Struthers
   D. Ulnar neuropathy below the elbow at the humeroulnar arcade

5. You are performing electrodiagnostic testing in a 29-year-old male with right digit 4 and 5 numbness and weakness. EMG testing so far shows 2+ positive sharp waves and fibrillation potentials in the first dorsal interosseous and the abductor digiti minimi. EMG testing of which muscle would be most helpful in distinguishing a C8 radiculopathy from an ulnar neuropathy?
   A. Pronator teres
   B. Flexor carpi ulnaris
   C. Palmaris brevis
   D. Extensor indicis proprius

Answers to the questions are located in Chapter 35.

REFERENCES

1. Landau ME, Campbell WW. Clinical features and electrodiagnosis of ulnar neuropathies [review]. *Phys Med Rehabil Clin N Am.* 2013;24(1):49–66. doi:10.1016/j.pmr.2012.08.019
2. Kincaid JC. AAEE minimonograph #31: the electrodiagnosis of ulnar neuropathy at the elbow. *Muscle Nerve.* 1988;11(10):1005–1015. doi:10.1002/mus.880111002

Radial Neuropathy

Jonathan S. Kirschner and Carlo Milani

INTRODUCTION

Radial neuropathy is commonly associated with lead poisoning (wrist drop), penetrating trauma and humeral fracture, sleeping with an arm slung around a chair or partner (Saturday night palsy, honeymooner's palsy), Wartenberg syndrome (superficial radial neuropathy at the elbow), posterior interosseous nerve (PIN) syndrome (compression about the elbow, neuralgic amyotrophy), and trauma or compression injury at the wrist ("cheiralgia paresthetica," handcuff neuropathy).

CLINICAL PRESENTATION

- Patients classically present with wrist drop, although depending on the site of the lesion one of four distinct syndromes may occur (Table 20.1).
- Patients present with mixed-motor and sensory symptoms in proximal lesions, but can present with pure motor or pure sensory complaints in distal lesions.
- Deltoid and latissimus weakness can help differentiate posterior cord lesions from proximal radial neuropathies. Preservation of triceps and brachioradialis (BR) reflexes helps rule out injury in the axilla and spiral groove, respectively. Pronator teres (PT) and flexor carpi ulnaris (FCU) weakness can differentiate C7 radiculopathy (1) from radial nerve injury.

Clinical Pearls

- *Tip:* Remember to test finger extension at the metacarpophalangeal joints with interphalangeal joints flexed to test the radial innervated extensor digitorum communis (EDC) and extensor indicis proprius (EIP); otherwise, you are testing median and ulnar innervated lumbricals.
- *Tip:* If the wrist and hand are not properly supported during examination, weakness of the wrist and finger extensors may cause apparent weakness of the finger flexors and abductors (median and ulnar distributions). During testing, weak wrist extensors may put the thumb and finger flexors at mechanical disadvantage (2), and weak finger extensors won't provide co-contraction needed to help intrinsic hand muscles function properly (3).

TABLE 20.1 Radial Neuropathy Syndromes

Injury Location	Muscles Affected	Weakness	Sensory Loss
Axilla (crutch palsy)	All radial muscles	Elbow extension, elbow flexion, wrist extension, finger extension, thumb extension and abduction	Posterior arm, dorsal forearm, dorsal hand
Spiral groove (Saturday night/honeymooner's palsy)	All but triceps, anconeus	Elbow flexion, wrist extension, finger extension, thumb extension and abduction	Dorsal hand
Supinator/arcade of Frohse (PIN syndrome)	All but triceps, anconeus, brachioradialis, extensor carpi radialis longus, extensor carpi radialis brevis	Ulnar deviated wrist extension, finger extension, thumb extension and abduction	None (pure motor injury)
Wrist (cheiralgia paresthetica)	None (pure sensory injury)	None (pure sensory injury)	Dorsal hand

PIN, posterior interosseous nerve.

ANATOMY

- The radial nerve is the mixed-motor and sensory terminal extension of the posterior cord of the brachial plexus after branches are given off to the axillary, thoracodorsal, and subscapular nerves (Figure 20.1).
- Fibers are derived from C5–T1 roots and the posterior divisions of all three trunks. Predominant dermatomal and myotomal contributions come from C5–C8 roots.
- In the upper arm, the radial nerve first branches into pure sensory nerves comprising the posterior cutaneous nerve of the arm, the lower lateral cutaneous nerve of the arm, and the posterior cutaneous nerve of the forearm.
- Motor branches are then given off to the anconeus and each head of the triceps before the nerve travels around the posterior humerus in the spiral groove.
- Branches are then given to the brachialis, BR, and extensor carpi radialis longus (ECR-L) above the lateral epicondyle. The extensor carpi radialis brevis (ECR-B) and supinator are supplied below the lateral epicondyle. The main radial trunk then bifurcates into a pure motor (PIN) and a pure sensory (superficial radial nerve [SRN]) branch.
- The PIN pierces the supinator and travels under the arcade of Frohse before supplying the remainder of the wrist and finger extensors. In some cases, the PIN may also supply the ECR-B and supinator.
- The SRN travels along the posterolateral forearm and supplies sensation to the dorsum of the hand and thumb, index, and middle and lateral half of the ring finger (except for the distal tips of the digits).

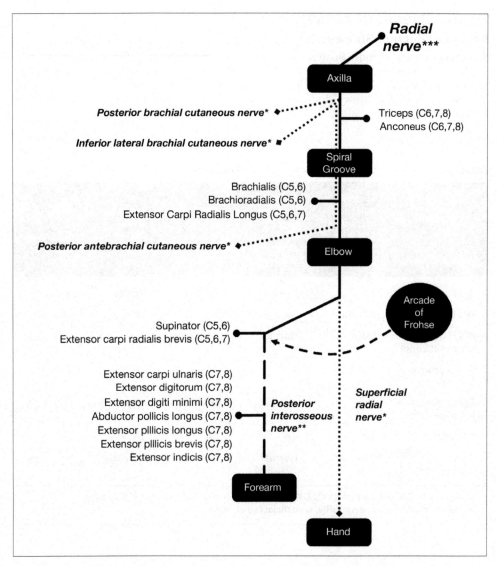

FIGURE 20.1 Schematic of the radial nerve; myotomes indicate predominate nerve root supply. *** Mixed-motor and sensory nerve, ** pure motor nerve, * pure sensory nerve.

ELECTRODIAGNOSTIC APPROACH
Nerve Conduction Studies

Typical evaluation includes bilateral SRN sensory studies (Table 20.2; Figure 20.2) with stimulation at the forearm, and radial nerve motor studies to the extensor indicis proprius (EIP) with stimulation at the forearm, below and above the spiral groove (Figure 20.3). Median and ulnar motor and sensory studies are usually performed for comparison and to rule out a more diffuse process.

TABLE 20.2 Nerve Conduction Studies in Radial Neuropathy

Location of Lesion	Sensory Nerve Response of SRN With Stimulation at Forearm	Motor Nerve Response Over EIP With Stimulation at Forearm	Stimulation at Arm Below Spiral Groove	Stimulation at Arm Above Spiral Groove	Stimulation at Erb's Point
SRN	↓A	Normal	Normal	Normal	Normal
PIN (axonal)	Normal	↓A	↓A	↓A	↓A
PIN (demyelinating)	Normal	Normal	↓CV ± CB	↓CV ± CB	↓CV ± CB
Spiral groove (axonal)	↓A	↓A	↓A	↓A	↓A
Spiral groove (demyelinating)	Normal	Normal	Normal	↓CV ± CB	↓CV ± CB
Axilla (axonal)	↓A	↓A	↓A	↓A	↓A
Axilla (demyelinating)	Normal	Normal	Normal	Normal	↓CV ± CB

A, amplitude; CB, conduction block; CV, conduction velocity; EIP, extensor indicis propius; PIN, posterior interosseous nerve; SRN, superficial radial nerve.

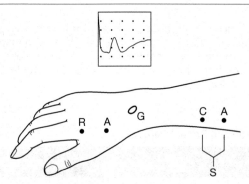

- A (active electrode): A 3-cm bar is placed with active electrode over the radial sensory nerve as it passes over the extensor pollicis longus tendon at the base of the first metacarpal.
- R (reference electrode): Is placed distal to the base of the thumb.
  - Alternatively, ring electrodes pick up over thumb.
- Stimulation site: (S) Cathode is placed 10 to 14 cm proximal, just over the radius laterally. Anode is proximal.
- Reference values obtained with bar electrode recording from dorsal hand: normal onset latency 1.9 ms, onset to peak amplitude 29 μV, conduction velocity 58 m/s, upper limit of amplitude difference side to side is approximately 60%.

FIGURE 20.2 Superficial radial nerve sensory conduction study.

Source: From Kumbhare D, Robinson L, Buschbacher R. *Manual of Nerve Conduction Studies*. 3rd ed. New York, NY: Demos Medical Publishing; 2015.

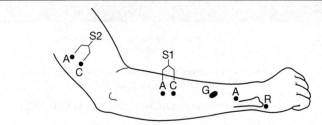

- A (active electrode): Is placed 4 cm proximal to ulnar styloid over motor point of EIP.
- R (reference electrode): Is over the ulnar styloid.
  - Alternatively, needle electrode is placed in EIP.
- Stimulation site: (S1) Cathode is 8 cm proximal to the electrode. Anode is proximal. (S2) Cathode is 8 to 10 cm proximal to the lateral epicondyle in the radial groove. Anode is proximal.
- Reference values obtained with bar electrode over EIP: Normal onset latency with forearm stimulation: 2.1 ms, onset to peak amplitude 4.5 mV, normal conduction velocity from above elbow (S2) to forearm (S1): 61.6 ± 5.9 m/s; normal conduction velocity from Erb's point to above elbow (S2): 72.0 ± 6.3 m/s.

FIGURE 20.3 Radial nerve motor conduction to extensor indicis proprius.

EIP, extensor indicis propius.

Source: From Kumbhare D, Robinson L, Buschbacher R. *Manual of Nerve Conduction Studies*. 3rd ed. New York, NY: Demos Medical Publishing; 2015.

Electromyography

A typical muscle screen needs to localize the lesion by testing above and below potential entrapment sites, including triceps or anconeus, BR, ECR-L, and extensor carpi ulnaris (ECU), EIP, or extensor digitorum communis (EDC). Posterior cord lesions should be assessed with deltoid or latissimus dorsi, and C7 radiculopathy with FCU, PT, or cervical paraspinals (Tables 20.3 and 20.4).

TABLE 20.3 EMG Screening in Radial Neuropathy

Helps Rule In Radial Neuropathy	Helps Rule Out Radial Neuropathy
Triceps or anconeus (axillary lesion)	Deltoid (C5, C6 radiculopathy, posterior cord)
Brachioradialis or extensor carpi radialis longus (spiral groove lesion)	Pronator teres (C6, C7 radiculopathy)
Extensor carpi ulnaris (PIN lesion)	Latissimus dorsi (C6, C7, C8 radiculopathy, posterior cord)
Extensor indicis proprius (distal PIN lesion)	Flexor carpi ulnaris (C7, C8 radiculopathy)
PIN, posterior interosseous nerve.	

TABLE 20.4 EMG Findings for Selected Injuries in Differential Diagnosis for Radial Neuropathy

Location of Lesion	Muscles Affected
C7 root	Cervical paraspinals, flexor carpi ulnaris, pronator teres, triceps, anconeus, ECR-L, ECU, EDC, EIP
Posterior cord	Deltoid, subscapularis, latissimus dorsi, triceps, anconeus, supinator, BR, ECR-L, ECU, EDC, EIP
Axilla	Triceps, anconeus, supinator, BR, ECR-L, ECU, EDC, EIP
Spiral groove	Supinator, BR, ECR-L, ECU, EDC, EIP
PIN	± Supinator, ECU, EDC, EIP

BR, brachioradialis; ECR-L, extensor carpi radialis longus; ECU, extensor carpi ulnaris; EDC, extensor digitorum communis; EIP, extensor indicis proprius; PIN, posterior interosseous nerve.

RECOVERY IN RADIAL NEUROPATHY

- Radial neuropathy is the most common peripheral nerve injury in upper extremity trauma, especially after humeral fracture (spiral groove).
- External compression injury is common [resting position, perioperative positioning (4)] and elbow arthroscopy (5) and Parsonage–Turner syndrome (6) are increasingly recognized sources of radial neuropathy.
- A majority of nontraumatic radial mononeuropathies achieve good functional recovery (7), and electrodiagnostic testing can facilitate prognostication (Table 20.5).
- In one study, electrodiagnostic features associated with good recovery included EIP motor response greater than 0.5 mV on nerve conduction studies, and any BR motor unit recruitment (8) on EMG (i.e., full, reduced, or discrete).
- In a separate study, normal posterior antebrachial cutaneous nerve (PACN) sensory response correlated with clinical improvement at 3 months, whereas PACN abnormality correlated with radial motor axon loss and a poorer prognosis (9).

TABLE 20.5 Electrodiagnostic Prognostic Indicators for Functional Recovery in Radial Neuropathy

Positive Indicators	Negative Indicators
BR motor unit recruitment full, reduced, or discrete	BR motor unit recruitment absent
EIP motor response >0.5 mV	EIP motor response <0.5 mV
PACN sensory response present	PACN sensory response absent
BR, brachioradialis; EIP, extensor indicis proprius; PACN, posterior antebrachial cutaneous nerve.	

QUESTIONS

1. A 28-year-old man presents to your office with left wrist drop 1 month following a gunshot wound to the upper arm. Abnormal spontaneous activity in which of the following muscles would differentiate posterior cord injury from an isolated radial nerve injury?
   A. Flexor carpi ulnaris
   B. Cervical paraspinals
   C. Latissimus dorsi
   D. Anconeus

Answers to the questions are located in Chapter 35.

2. You perform needle EMG on the same patient and obtain the following results:

Muscle	Insertional Activity	Fibrillation Potential	Positive Sharp Wave	Fasciculation	Amplitude	Duration	Recruitment
Deltoid	nl	0	0	0	nl	nl	nl
Triceps	nl	0	0	0	nl	nl	nl
Brachioradialis	nl	0	0	0	nl	nl	nl
Extensor carpi radialis longus	↓	2+	2+	0	nl	nl	↓
Extensor indicis proprius	↓	3+	3+	0	nl	nl	↓
Flexor carpi ulnaris	nl	0	0	0	nl	nl	nl
Pronator teres	nl	0	0	0	nl	nl	nl
Paraspinals	nl	0	0	0	nl	nl	nl

nl, normal.

The lesion is most likely:
A. At the nerve root
B. At the posterior cord
C. At the axilla
D. Below the spiral groove
E. Below the lateral epicondyle
F. In the arcade of Frohse

3. You perform needle EMG on another patient and obtain the following results:

Muscle	Insertional Activity	Fibrillation Potential	Positive Sharp Wave	Fasciculation	Amplitude	Duration	Recruitment
Deltoid	↓	1+	1+	0	nl	nl	↓
Triceps	nl	0	0	0	nl	nl	nl
Brachioradialis	nl	0	0	0	nl	nl	nl
Extensor carpi radialis longus	↓	2+	2+	0	nl	nl	↓
Extensor indicis proprius	↓	3+	3+	0	nl	nl	↓
Flexor carpi ulnaris	nl	0	0	0	nl	nl	nl
Pronator teres	nl	0	0	0	nl	nl	nl
Paraspinals	nl	0	0	0	nl	nl	nl

nl, normal.

The lesion is most likely:
A. At the nerve root
B. At the posterior cord
C. At the axilla
D. Below the spiral groove
E. Below the lateral epicondyle
F. In the arcade of Frohse

4. You perform needle EMG on another patient and obtain the following results:

Muscle	Insertional Activity	Fibrillation Potential	Positive Sharp Wave	Fasciculation	Amplitude	Duration	Recruitment
Deltoid	nl	0	0	0	nl	nl	nl
Triceps	↓	2+	2+	0	nl	nl	↓
Brachioradialis	nl	0	0	0	nl	nl	nl
Extensor carpi radialis longus	↓	2+	2+	0	nl	nl	↓
Extensor indicis proprius	nl	0	0	0	nl	nl	nl
Flexor carpi ulnaris	↓	1+	1+	0	nl	nl	↓
Pronator teres	nl	0	0	0	nl	nl	nl
Paraspinals	↓	1+	1+	0	nl	nl	↓

nl, normal.

The lesion is most likely:
A. At the nerve root
B. At the posterior cord
C. In the axilla
D. Below the spiral groove
E. Below the lateral epicondyle
F. In the arcade of Frohse

5. A 46-year-old man presents with a 2-month history of wrist drop after passing out on a park bench following a prolonged drinking session. You suspect an axonotmetic radial nerve injury at the spiral groove. On electrodiagnostic testing, you would expect to find:
A. A normal superficial sensory nerve action potential
B. Abnormal spontaneous activity in the anconeus
C. A normal compound muscle action potential with stimulation at the forearm and recording over the extensor indicis proprius
D. Abnormal spontaneous activity in the brachioradialis

6. A 39-year-old man presents with a 2-month history of slowly progressive weakness in the right wrist and finger extensors. Prior to the weakness, he was woken from sleep by a severe pain in the right shoulder and forearm that resolved after 3 days. He denies sensory deficits. Past medical history includes recovery from a viral illness 3 months ago and a contusion to the right dorsal forearm while playing with his toddler. The most likely cause of his symptoms is:

   A. Cervical radiculopathy
   B. Humeral fracture
   C. Parsonage–Turner syndrome (neuralgic amyotrophy)
   D. Compressive hematoma
   E. Superficial radial neuropathy
   F. Wartenberg syndrome

ADDITIONAL READINGS

Date ES, Teraoka JK, Chan J, et al. Effects of elbow flexion on radial nerve motor conduction velocity. *Electromyogr Clin Neurophysiol*. 2002;42:51–66. PubMed PMID: 11851010.

Jebsen, R. Motor conduction velocity in proximal and distal segments of the radial nerve. *Arch Phys Med Rehabil*. 1966;47:597–602. PubMed PMID: 5919251.

Trojaborg W, Sindrup EH. Motor and sensory conduction in different segments of the radial nerve. *J Neurol Neurosurg Psychiatr*. 1969;32:354–359. doi:10.1136/jnnp.32.4.354

REFERENCES

1. Pyun SB, Kang S, Kwon HK. Anatomical and electrophysiological myotomes corresponding to the flexor carpi ulnaris muscle. *J Korean Med Sci*. 2010;25(3):454–457. doi:10.3346/jkms.2010.25.3.454
2. Labosky DA, Waggy CA. Apparent weakness of median and ulnar motors in radial nerve palsy. *J Hand Surg Am*. 1986;11(4):528–533. doi:10.1016/s0363-5023(86)80191-5
3. Sadeh M, Gilad R, Dabby R, et al. Apparent weakness of ulnar-innervated muscles in radial palsy. *Neurology*. 2004;62(8):1424–1425. doi:10.1212/01.wnl.0000120666.08352.72
4. Tuncali BE, Tuncali B, Kuvaki B, et al. Radial nerve injury after general anaesthesia in the lateral decubitus position. *Anaesthesia*. 2005;60(6):602–604. doi:10.1111/j.1365-2044.2005.04177.x
5. Desai MJ, Mithani SK, Lodha SJ, et al. Major peripheral nerve injuries after elbow arthroscopy. *Arthroscopy*. 2016;32(6):999–1002.e1008. doi:10.1016/j.arthro.2015.11.023
6. Milner CS, Kannan K, Iyer VG, et al. Parsonage-Turner syndrome: clinical and epidemiological features from a hand surgeon's perspective. *Hand (NY)*. 2016;11(2):227–231. doi:10.1177/1558944715627246
7. Bsteh G, Wanschitz JV, Gruber H, et al. Prognosis and prognostic factors in non-traumatic acute-onset compressive mononeuropathies—radial and peroneal mononeuropathies. *Eur J Neurol*. 2013;20(6):981–985. doi:10.1111/ene.12150
8. Malikowski T, Micklesen PJ, Robinson LR. Prognostic values of electrodiagnostic studies in traumatic radial neuropathy. *Muscle Nerve*. 2007;36(3):364–367. doi:10.1002/mus.20848
9. Lo YL, Prakash KM, Leoh TH, et al. Posterior antebrachial cutaneous nerve conduction study in radial neuropathy. *J Neurol Sci*. 2004;223(2):199–202. doi:10.1016/j.jns.2004.05.004

21

Anterior Interosseous Nerve Lesions

Patrick J. Barrett

INTRODUCTION

Anterior interosseous nerve (AIN) lesions occur rarely; they are also known as *Kiloh–Nevin syndrome*. It is especially important to be aware of the clinical presentation and common anomalies to detect its presence, as the basic nerve conduction studies (NCS) are often normal.

ANATOMY

- The AIN emanates from C5–T1 roots, medial and lateral cord of brachial plexus, and median nerve just distal to the pronator teres muscle (typically 5–8 cm distal to lateral epicondyle) in the forearm. It is the largest branch of the median nerve.
- There is no cutaneous innervation, though there are sensory fibers to the wrist and interosseous membrane.
- It provides innervation to three muscles: the flexor pollicis longus (FPL), pronator quadratus, and the flexor digitorum profundus to digits 2 and 3.

PATHOPHYSIOLOGY

- Several etiologies of AIN neuropathy have been described, including an entrapment due to compression from an anomalous fibrous band or an accessory head of the FPL (Gantzer muscle), neuralgic amyotrophy, lacerations, gunshot wounds, fractures, pregnancy, and muscular exertion (1–8).

CLINICAL PRESENTATION

- Typically, patients with AIN lesions complain of an inability to pick up objects with the thumb and index finger.
  - The AIN has no cutaneous sensory fibers; thus, there should be no sensory complaints. However, some patients complain of a dull ache in the forearm, especially early in the course (9,10).
- Physical examination reveals weakness in the AIN-innervated muscles: the pronator quadratus, the FPL, and the FDP to the 2nd and 3rd digits.

- To isolate pronator quadratus muscle strength on physical examination, pronation should be tested when the elbow is flexed to reduce pronation from the pronator teres muscle.
- In addition, patients with AIN injuries will not be able to make an "OK" sign with their thumb and 2nd digit. Instead of the tips of their fingers touching, the volar surfaces of the fingers will be in contact secondary to the weakness of the FPL and the FDP muscles (Figure 21.1).
- Sensory and reflex examinations should be normal.

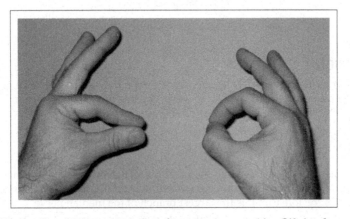

FIGURE 21.1 OK sign: The right is normal; the left represents a positive OK sign for an anterior interosseous nerve lesion affecting both the flexor pollicis longus and the flexor digitorum profundus. Clinically, a complete lesion like this is uncommon.

ELECTRODIAGNOSTIC APPROACH

- Differential diagnosis of weakness in AIN-innervated muscles besides an injury to AIN includes more proximal median nerve injuries, brachial plexopathies, radiculopathies, and polyneuropathies.
- A well-designed electrodiagnostic study should investigate for these possibilities.
- Recommended nerve conduction studies that should be performed:
  - Routine median and ulnar sensory and motor studies. These studies should be normal in isolated AIN lesions.
  - In addition to the routine tests, a median motor test may be performed by recording over the pronator quadratus. The active electrode is placed on the dorsal forearm, 3 cm proximal to the ulna styloid between the radius and the ulna. The reference electrode is placed on the ulna styloid.
    - Compound muscle action potential (CMAP) baseline-to-peak amplitude is 3.1 + 0.8 mV (2.0–5.5 mV).

- ☐ Side-to-side comparison acceptable difference is less than 25%.
- ☐ CMAP onset latency is 3.6 + 0.4 ms (2.9–4.4 ms), with side-to-side comparison acceptable difference being less than 0.4 ms (11).
- Needle EMG should always be performed:
  - At least the three muscles innervated by the AIN (i.e., FDP, FPL, and pronator quadratus) should be examined to assess for muscle membrane instability (see Table 21.1 for landmarks).
  - More proximal median-innervated muscles should also be assessed to rule out a more proximal median entrapment, and other muscles should also be tested to rule out a cervical radiculopathy or brachial plexopathy.

TABLE 21.1 Landmarks for Muscles Innervated by the Anterior Interosseous Nerve

Muscle	Landmarks
Flexor digitorum profundus	The tip of the little finger is placed on the olecranon. The ring, middle, and index fingers are placed along the shaft of the ulna. The electrode is inserted just beyond the index finger and just ulnar to the shaft. The median-innervated portion lies deeper.
Flexor pollicis longus	The electrode is inserted in the middle of the forearm at the apex of the antecubital fossa. Insert electrode until bone is reached and then pull back slightly. Flexor pollicis longus is the last muscle before the bone.
Pronator quadratus	Patient's arm is placed at the side, supinated with the wrist flexed. The electrode is inserted just anterior to the distal aspect of the ulnar shaft. The electrode is then advanced horizontally into the muscle belly. Using this medial approach avoids the median nerve that lies ventrally.

Source: From Geiringer SR. *Anatomic Localization for Needle Electromyography.* 2nd ed. Philadelphia, PA: Hanley & Belfus; 1999.

- Special considerations/presentations:
  - An AIN injury in those patients with a Martin–Gruber anastomosis may be difficult to determine.
    - ☐ A Martin–Gruber anastomosis is a median-to-ulnar crossover of fibers, and these fibers are commonly found in the AIN.
    - ☐ Abnormalities may also be seen in the ulnar-innervated intrinsic muscles of the hand, such as the first dorsal interosseous muscle, adductor pollicis, and abductor digiti minimi (12). These muscles should also be checked with needle EMG if a Martin–Gruber anastomosis is suspected.

QUESTIONS

1. What sign is used to test for an anterior interosseous nerve injury?
   A. Froment sign
   B. Wartenberg sign
   C. OK sign
   D. Piano key sign

2. Choose the best way to examine pronator quadratus strength on physical examination.
   A. Pronation when the wrist is flexed
   B. Pronation when the wrist is extended
   C. Pronation when the elbow is flexed
   D. Pronation when the elbow is extended

3. Patients with anterior interosseous nerve injury have loss of sensation in what distribution?
   A. C7 distribution
   B. Palmar branch of the median nerve distribution
   C. Dorsal ulnar cutaneous distribution
   D. There is no loss of cutaneous sensation

4. Patients with a Martin–Gruber anastomosis who sustain an anterior interosseous nerve injury may also demonstrate weakness in which muscle?
   A. Flexor digitorum superficialis
   B. Adductor pollicis
   C. Pronator teres
   D. Abductor pollicis brevis

REFERENCES

1. Brussé CA, Burke FD. Recurrent anterior interosseous nerve palsies related to pregnancy. *J Hand Surg Br.* 1998;23(1):102–103. PubMed PMID: 9571495.
2. Farber JS, Bryan RS. The anterior interosseous nerve syndrome. *J Bone Joint Surg Am.* 1968;50(3):521–523. PubMed PMID: 5644869.
3. Griffiths JC. Nerve injuries after plating of forearm bones. *Br Med J.* 1966;2(5508):277–279. PubMed PMID: 5945556.
4. Hill NA, Howard FM, Huffer BR. The incomplete anterior interosseous nerve syndrome. *J Hand Surg Am.* 1985;10(1):4–16. PubMed PMID: 3968404.
5. Matsuzaki A, Kobayashi A, Misuyasu M, Morooka M, Honda K. 5 Cases of neuralgic amyotrophy with neuroparalysis of the anterior interosseous nerve as a main symptom [in Japanese]. *Seikei Geka.* 1969;20(8):916–923. PubMed PMID: 5817526.
6. Megele R. Anterior interosseous nerve syndrome with atypical nerve course in relation to the pronator teres. *Acta Neurochir (Wien).* 1988;91(3–4):144–146. PubMed PMID: 3407460.
7. Rennels GD, Ochoa J. Neuralgic amyotrophy manifesting as anterior interosseous nerve palsy. *Muscle Nerve.* 1980;3(2):160–164. doi:10.1002/mus.880030209

Answers to the questions are located in Chapter 35.

8. Spinner M, Schreiber SN. Anterior interosseous-nerve paralysis as a complication of supracondylar fractures of the humerus in children. *J Bone Joint Surg Am.* 1969;51(8): 1584–1590. PubMed PMID: 5357177.
9. Schmidt H, Eiken O. The anterior interosseous nerve syndrome. Case reports. *Scand J Plast Reconstr Surg.* 1971;5:53–56. PubMed PMID: 5559733.
10. Spinner M. The anterior interosseous nerve syndrome: With special attention to its variations. *J Bone Joint Surg Am.* 1970;52:84–94. PubMed PMID: 5411776.
11. Dumitru D, Zwarts MJ. Focal peripheral neuropathies. In: Dumitru D, Amato AA, Zwarts MJ, eds. *Electrodiagnostic Medicine.* 2nd ed. Philadelphia, PA: Hanley & Belfus; 2002:1057–1058.
12. Mannerfelt L. Studies on the hand in ulnar nerve paralysis. A clinical-experimental investigation in normal and anomalous innervation. *Acta Orthop Scand.* 1996;(suppl 87):1. PubMed PMID: 4287179.

22

Fibular (Peroneal) Neuropathy

Rohini Sweta Rao and Aaron Jay Yang

INTRODUCTION
The common fibular nerve is one of the two nerves (along with the tibial nerve) that make up the sciatic nerve. The common fibular nerve, and its branches, the superficial and deep fibular nerves, are far more commonly referred to by their older name (the *peroneal nerves*); however, in keeping with modern nomenclature, we will use the term *fibular nerve*. The most common clinical presentation of fibular neuropathy is foot drop and/or sensory changes over the lateral aspect of the calf and dorsum of the foot. Nerve conduction studies and electromyography have proven to be crucial in the identification and localization of the level of injury.

CLINICAL PRESENTATION
- The most common site of intraneural ganglia within the peripheral nervous system is around the common fibular nerve. Fibular nerve compromise has been reported due to numerous traumatic and insidious causes and can be broken down into the categories of trauma, stretch, compression, entrapment, mass lesions, and miscellaneous.
  - Trauma
    - Proximal fibular and tibial fractures
    - Isolated nerve laceration
    - Isolated nerve traction
      - Ankle sprain, nerve fixed proximally at the fibular head, nerve fixed distally at the extensor retinaculum, and nerve stretched by rapid ankle plantarflexion and inversion
    - Ligamentous knee injury, particularly the anterior cruciate ligament
  - Compression
    - Casting material at the fibular head, anterior compartment of the leg, or extensor retinaculum
    - Operative positioning causing compression at the fibular head
  - Insidious causes
    - Mass lesions and metabolic syndromes
  - Miscellaneous
    - Knee arthrodesis, total knee arthroplasty, realignment of the knee extensor mechanism, and arthroscopic meniscal repair

160 | Common Clinical Entities

- Key elements on physical examination:
  - Sensory examination (Figure 22.1)
    - ☐ Sensation changes in the mid and lower lateral calf and dorsum of the foot between digits 1 and 2 as these are supplied by the deep fibular nerve
    - ☐ Lateral and plantar foot regions are spared in lesions of the fibular nerve

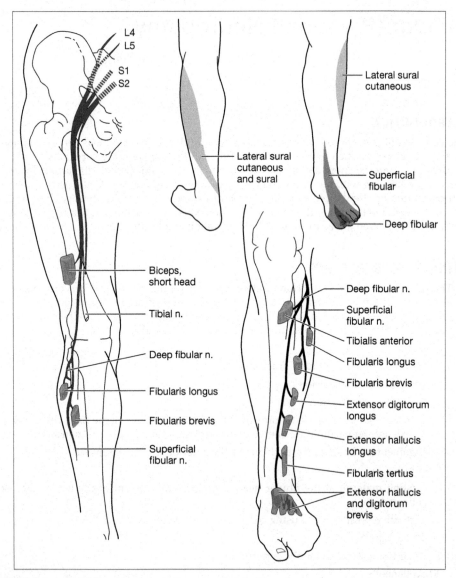

FIGURE 22.1 Anatomy of the peroneal nerve.

Source: Adapted from Jenkins DB. *Hollinshead's Functional Anatomy of the Limbs and Back.* 8th ed. Philadelphia, PA: WB Saunders; 2002.

- Motor examination
  - Foot drop is the most common presenting symptom
    - Weakness in foot dorsiflexion due to deep peroneal nerve innervation disruption
    - Weakness in foot eversion due to superficial peroneal nerve innervation disruption
  - Inversion and plantar flexion of the foot is preserved as these are innervated by the posterior tibial nerve
  - Table 22.1 provides a complete list of causes of foot drop

TABLE 22.1 Potential Causes for Foot Drop

Nerve	L5	Lumbosacral Plexopathy Variable Presentation: Example Is Lesion Proximal to Sciatic Nerve	Sciatic Nerve	Common Fibular Nerve	Deep Fibular Nerve	Superficial Fibular Nerve
Sensory changes	Lateral leg, lateral calf, dorsum of foot and medial toes	Posterior thigh, lateral calf, dorsal and plantar foot (sparing lateral foot)	Lateral calf, dorsal and plantar foot (sparing lateral foot)	Lateral calf and dorsum of foot (sparing lateral and plantar foot)	Area between great and second toes	Lateral calf and dorsum of foot (sparing lateral foot)
Motor Groups Affected						
Gluteus maximus	X					
Gluteus medius	X	X				
Gluteus minimus	X	X				
Tensor fascia latae	X	X				
Semitendinosus	X	X	X			
Semimembranosus	X	X	X			
Biceps femoris	X	X	X			

(continued)

TABLE 22.1 Potential Causes for Foot Drop (*continued*)

Nerve	L5	Lumbosacral Plexopathy Variable Presentation: Example Is Lesion Proximal to Sciatic Nerve	Sciatic Nerve	Common Fibular Nerve	Deep Fibular Nerve	Superficial Fibular Nerve
Tibialis posterior	X	X	X			
Tibialis anterior	X	X	X	X	X	
Peroneus longus	X	X	X	X		X
Peroneus brevis	X	X	X	X		X
Peroneus tertius		X	X	X	X	
Flexor digitorum brevis		X	X			
Flexor digitorum longus			X			
Flexor hallucis brevis		X	X			
Extensor digitorum brevis	X	X	X	X	X	
Extensor digitorum longus		X	X	X	X	
Extensor hallucis brevis		X	X	X	X	
Extensor hallucis longus	X	X		X	X	
Abductor digiti minimi		X	X			

(*continued*)

TABLE 22.1 Potential Causes for Foot Drop (*continued*)

Nerve	L5	Lumbosacral Plexopathy Variable Presentation: Example Is Lesion Proximal to Sciatic Nerve	Sciatic Nerve	Common Fibular Nerve	Deep Fibular Nerve	Superficial Fibular Nerve
Adductor hallucis		X	X			
Interossei		X	X			
Gastrocnemius		X				
Soleus		X				
Associated Weakness						
Hip abduction	X	X				
Hip internal rotation	X	X				
Partial hip adduction		X	X			
Knee flexion	X	X	X			
Ankle dorsiflexion	X	X	X	X	X	
Ankle plantar flexion		X	X			
Ankle inversion	X	X	X			
Ankle eversion	X	X	X	X		X
Toe extension	X	X	X	X	X	

- Anatomy
  - The sciatic nerve, the largest nerve in the body, receives its contributions from L4–S3.
  - The sciatic nerve divides into the common fibular nerve and the tibial nerves proximal to the posterior fossa.

- The common fibular nerve innervates the following before splitting into the deep and superficial fibular nerves just distal to the head of the fibula.
  - ☐ The short head of biceps femoris
  - ☐ The lateral sensory aspect of the leg via the lateral cutaneous nerve
- The deep fibular nerve innervates the following:
  - Anterior muscles of the leg—tibialis anterior, extensor digitorum longus, fibularis (peroneus) tertius, and extensor hallucis longus
  - Short toe extensors of the foot—extensor digitorum brevis (EDB), extensor hallucis brevis, and the intertarsal joints
  - Cutaneous branch for the web space between the 1st and 2nd toes
- The superficial fibular nerve innervates:
  - Fibularis (peroneus) longus and brevis
  - Sensation to the skin of the lateral leg as well as the dorsum of the foot and toes with the exception of the small area between the first two toes and a variable lateral part of the foot
- Accessory fibular (peroneal) nerve:
  - Seen in approximately 20% of patients
  - When present, it is a branch of the superficial fibular nerve that passes posteriorly to the lateral malleolus
  - It supplies the EDB (usually innervated by the deep fibular nerve)
  - In cases where stimulation of the fibular nerve at the ankle yields a smaller compound muscle action potential (CMAP) than that obtained on proximal stimulation, there may be an accessory fibular nerve
  - If stimulation posterior to the lateral malleolus results in a similar waveform to the proximal fibular motor studies, an accessory fibular nerve is present

ELECTRODIAGNOSTIC APPROACH

- Motor nerve conduction studies
  - Fibular nerve conduction study:
    - ☐ Recording electrode (A) is placed over the EDB on the dorsum of the foot
    - ☐ Reference electrode (B) is placed over the metacarpophalangeal joint of the 5th digit
    - ☐ The stimulator is placed 8 cm more proximal from the recording electrode slightly lateral to the tibialis anterior tendon
    - ☐ Ground electrode is placed on the dorsum of the foot (Figure 22.2)

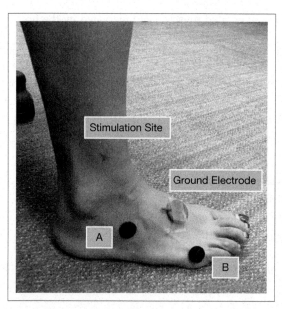

FIGURE 22.2 Placement of recording electrode (A) and reference electrode (B).

- Proximal stimulation should occur below the fibular head and 10 cm proximal to that in the lateral popliteal fossa.
- Performing a tibialis anterior study can be useful when the lesion is between the branches supplying the tibialis anterior and the EDB as well as for comorbid diseases (e.g., diabetic peripheral neuropathy) that cause atrophy of the distal EDB muscle.
- Tibial, sural, and fibular nerve studies must also be done to exclude more proximal lesions. These are described in their respective chapters.
  - If these studies are borderline, comparison should be made to the unaffected limb same day.
- Sensory nerve conduction studies of the superficial fibular nerve
  - Electrode is placed over the proximal ankle between the tibialis anterior tendon and lateral malleolus.
  - Stimulator is placed 14 cm proximally.
- Needle EMG
  - Important for the confirmation of localization assessment of severity of lesion; and exclusion of sciatic neuropathy, lumbosacral plexopathy, or radiculopathy
    - Two muscles innervated by the deep fibular nerve (e.g., tibialis anterior and extensor hallucis longus)
    - One muscle innervated by the superficial fibular nerve (fibularis longus and fibularis brevis)

- ☐ A group of L5-innervated muscles *not* innervated by the fibular nerve (e.g., tibialis posterior)
- ☐ A muscle innervated by the tibial nerve (e.g., medial gastrocnemius, soleus, flexor digitorum longus)
- ☐ The short head of the biceps femoris (the only muscle innervated by the common fibular nerve, and the only fibular-innervated muscle proximal to the knee)

QUESTIONS

1. What is the sensory distribution of the deep fibular nerve?
   A. Anterolateral shin
   B. Anterolateral shin and dorsum of the foot
   C. Dorsum of the foot
   D. Between the great toe and the second toe

2. What condition(s) cause(s) sensory and motor deficits similar to common fibular neuropathy?
   A. Sciatic neuropathy
   B. L5 radiculopathy
   C. Tibial neuropathy
   D. Both A and B

3. Where do you place the stimulator to determine whether there is an accessory fibular nerve?
   A. On the dorsum of the foot over the tendon of the extensor hallucis longus
   B. Anterior to the lateral malleolus
   C. Posterior to the lateral malleolus
   D. Anterior to the medial malleolus

4. Common fibular nerve innervates which muscle/muscle groups directly before splitting into the deep and superficial branches?
   A. Tibialis anterior, extensor digitorum longus, fibularis tertius, extensor hallucis longus
   B. Extensor digitorum brevis, extensor hallucis brevis, and tarsal joints
   C. Short head of biceps femoris
   D. Peroneus longus and peroneus brevis

Answers to the questions are located in Chapter 35.

5. What should be done in any conduction or EMG study that is abnormal or borderline when testing for peroneal neuropathy?
   A. Repeat study should be done on the affected side same day
   B. Repeat study should be done on the unaffected side same day
   C. Repeat study should be done on the affected side in 3 months
   D. Repeat study should be done on the unaffected side in 3 months

6. Weakness with which maneuver would NOT indicate a common peroneal nerve injury?
   A. Ankle dorsiflexion
   B. Ankle eversion
   C. Toe extension
   D. Ankle inversion

ADDITIONAL READINGS

Baima J, Krivickas L. Evaluation and treatment of peroneal neuropathy. *Curr Rev Musculoskelet Med.* 2008;1(2):147–153. doi:10.1007/s12178-008-9023-6

Dimitru D. Focal peripheral neuropathies. In: *Electrodiagnostic Medicine*. Philadelphia, PA: Hanley and Belfus; 1995:898.

Fetzer GB, Prather H, Gelberman RH, et al. Progressive fibular nerve palsy in a varus arthritic knee. A case report. *J Bone Joint Surg Am.* 2004;86-A(7):1538–1540. PubMed PMID: 15252107.

Katirji MB, Wilbourn AJ. Common fibular mononeuropathy: a clinical and electrophysiologic study of 116 lesions. *Neurology*. 1988;38:1723–1728. PubMed PMID: 2847078.

Kim DH, Murovic JA, Teil RL, et al. Management and outcomes in 318 operative common fibular nerve lesions at the LSU Health Sciences Center. *Neurosurgery*. 2004;54:1421–1429. PubMed PMID: 15157299.

Preston DC, Shapiro BE. Electromyography and neuromuscular disorders. *Fibular Neuropathy*. Philadelphia, PA: Elsevier; 2005:343–354.

Spinner RJ, Atkinson JL, Tiel RL. Fibular intraneural ganglia: the importance of the articular branch. A unifying theory. *J Neurosurg.* 2003;99:330–343. doi:10.3171/jns.2003.99.2.0330

Van Langenhove M, Pollefliet A, Vanderstraeten G. A retrospective electrodiagnostic evaluation of footdrop in 303 patients. *Electromyogr Clin Neurophysiol.* 1989;29:145–152. PubMed PMID: 2721427.

Tibial Neuropathy

Brian F. White

INTRODUCTION

In general, lower limb peripheral nerve injuries are much less common than those involving the upper limb and comprise approximately 25% of identified peripheral nerve injuries (1). Among lower limb nerves, the fibular (peroneal) and tibial nerves are commonly involved in nerve injury and neuropathy. The tibial nerve may be compromised in tarsal tunnel syndrome due to trauma or compression. Along its course in the lower limb, the tibial nerve may also be involved in various forms of neuropathy.

CLINICAL PRESENTATION

Clinical presentation will vary depending on both the type and anatomic location of injury. Given its length, diverse course, and the varied anatomic distribution it serves, tibial nerve lesions present with a heterogeneous set of findings.

- Tarsal tunnel: Common findings will include burning or tingling pain in the sole of the involved foot (2).
- Proximal injuries may present with sensory symptoms in the foot, similar to tarsal tunnel syndrome, as well as posterior calf symptoms in the distribution of the medial sural cutaneous nerve.
- Motor involvement will depend on the level of the lesion and may present with weakness in ankle plantar flexion and inversion and possibly knee flexion. Multiple entrapment sites have been described (Table 23.1).
- Achilles reflex may be reduced in proximal lesions (Table 23.2).

BASIC ANATOMY

- The tibial nerve is derived from the ventral rami of the L4–S3 and exits the pelvis at the sciatic foramen as a bundled portion of the sciatic nerve.
- It courses distally in the posterior thigh as the medial division of the sciatic nerve bundled within the sciatic nerve sheath along with lateral division, which becomes the peroneal nerve. The two divisions separate into their respective named nerves several centimeters proximal to the knee.

- The tibial nerve proper courses distally through the popliteal space and into the posterior calf. Just distal to the knee, the tibial nerve lies deep to the gastrocnemius muscle and superficial to the popliteus muscle in the midline. At the inferior margin of the popliteus muscle, the tibial nerve dives deep through the tendinous arch of the soleus muscle and then continues within the deep posterior compartment of the leg distally to the medial ankle.
- Posterior to the medial malleolus, the tibial nerve passes beneath the medial flexor retinaculum within the tarsal tunnel and divides into its three terminal branches: the medial calcaneal, medial plantar, and lateral plantar nerves.
- Motor innervation is reviewed in Table 23.3.
- Sensory innervation is reviewed in Table 23.4.

TABLE 23.1 Tibial Nerve Entrapment or Injury Sites

Site	Notes
Trauma	Traumatic injury may occur at any point along the course of the tibial nerve or to tibial fibers within the sciatic nerve.
Popliteal fossa	Tibial nerve may be compressed by mass such as a Baker cyst.
Tendinous arch of soleus	Nerve may be compressed by the fibers of the arch of the soleus as the nerve enters the deep compartment of the leg.
Deep posterior compartment	Compartment syndrome occurs in the deep compartment.
Tarsal tunnel	Nerve may be compressed under medial flexor retinaculum.

TABLE 23.2 Reflexes

Reflex	Components
Achilles reflex	Both afferent and efferent portions of the reflex arc travel on the tibial nerve.

TABLE 23.3 Tibial Motor Innervation

Location	Significant Muscles
Proximal to knee	• Four muscles: the long head of biceps femoris, semimembranosus, semitendinosus, and the posterior portion of the adductor magnus
Knee to tarsal tunnel	• Seven muscles: plantaris, gastrocnemius, popliteus, soleus, tibialis posterior, flexor digitorum longus, flexor hallucis longus
Distal to tarsal tunnel	• Via the medial plantar nerve: abductor hallucis, flexor digitorum brevis, flexor hallucis brevis • Via the lateral plantar nerve: abductor digiti quinti

TABLE 23.4 Tibial Sensory Innervation

Location	Sensory Nerves
Proximal to knee	• Medial sural nerve, which joins with the peroneal-derived sural communicating branch to form the sural nerve in the lateral calf; this provides sensation to the lateral aspect of the calf as well as the lateral margin of the posterior half of the foot
Knee to tarsal tunnel	• Medial articular branch to the knee and the sensory interosseous nerve
Distal to tarsal tunnel	• Via the medial plantar nerve: medial sole of the foot, medial 3½ toes, analogous to the finger innervation by the median nerve • Via the lateral plantar nerve: lateral sole of the foot, lateral 1½ toes, analogous to the finger innervation by the ulnar nerve • Via the calcaneal nerve: skin overlying the heel pad, analogous to the palmar cutaneous branch of the median nerve in the hand

ELECTRODIAGNOSTIC APPROACH

There are a variety of approaches to the evaluation of a potential tibial nerve lesion or neuropathy. Many sensory, motor, and mixed nerve conduction studies (NCS) are described, several of which are included here. The appropriate studies to use in patient evaluation will depend on many factors, with clinical presentation and the suspected clinical differential diagnosis being driving forces in the choice of conduction studies as well as the specific decisions regarding needle EMG.

- Sensory evaluation should include either medial or lateral plantar NCS, depending on the location of clinical symptoms. Sensory evaluation should also include sural sensory as well as superficial fibular (peroneal) sensory NCS (Chapters 7 and 22); see Table 23.5 for full description. The contralateral limb should also be studied for comparison.
- Motor evaluation should include the tibial motor NCS to abductor hallucis, with stimulation at the medial ankle and proximally at the popliteal fossa; see Table 23.6 for full description. An abnormal study requires additional study of both the ipsilateral deep fibular (peroneal) motor NCS to the extensor digitorum brevis (EDB; Chapter 6) and the tibial motor NCS on the contralateral side.
- Mixed-nerve studies may be alternatively used depending on physician preference; see Table 23.7 for a full description.
- Delayed responses include tibial F-wave (Chapter 8) and H-reflex (Chapter 9). These studies may highlight proximal demyelination or focal demyelination at a site of compression (Table 23.8).

TABLE 23.5 Tibial Sensory Nerve Conduction Studies

Name	Lead Placement	Stimulation Site	Normal Values
Medial plantar sensory (orthodromic study)	• E1: Posterior to and slightly proximal from the medial malleolus; positioned just proximal to the flexor retinaculum • E2: 4 cm proximal to E1	Ring electrodes placed on the great toe with cathode proximal and anode distal; distance will be variable to each individual	• Distal onset latency: Not measured • Amplitude: ≥2.0 μV • Conduction velocity: ≥35 m/s
Lateral plantar sensory (orthodromic study)	• E1 and E2 placed same as described for medial plantar nerve	Ring electrodes placed on the little toe with cathode proximal and anode distal	• Distal onset latency: Not measured • Amplitude: ≥1.0 μV • Conduction velocity: ≥35 m/s
Sural sensory	• E1: Posterior to the lateral malleolus, 1 cm proximal from the tip of the fibula • E2: 4 cm distal to E1	Calf: 14 cm proximal to E1 in the posterior lateral calf	• Distal onset latency: ≤4.4 ms • Amplitude: ≥6 μV • Conduction velocity: >40 m/s

Source: From Preston DC, Shapiro BE. Routine lower extremity nerve conduction techniques. In: *Electromyography and Neuromuscular Disorders: Clinical–Electrophysiologic Correlations.* 3rd ed. New York, NY: Elsevier Saunders; 2013:115–124.

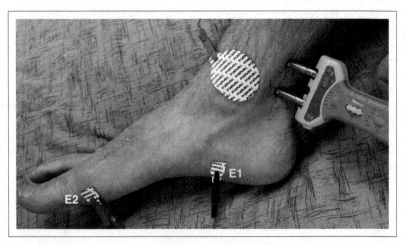

FIGURE 23.1 Tibial motor nerve conduction studies setup to AH. E1 (black): Placed over muscle belly of AH. E2 (gray): Placed over the metatarsophalangeal of the great toe.

AH, abductor hallucis.

TABLE 23.6 Tibial Motor Nerve Conduction Studies

Name	Lead Placement	Stimulation Site	Normal Values
Tibial motor to AH Tests medial plantar nerve terminal division	• E1: Over muscle belly of AH, 1 cm inferior and 1 cm proximal to the navicular prominence • E2: Placed more distally, over the metatarsophalangeal of the great toe	• Ankle: Posterior to the medial malleolus, 8 cm proximal from E1 • Knee: Midline in the popliteal fossa, between the two heads of the gastrocnemius	• Distal onset latency: <6.1 ms • Side-to-side difference: <1.4 ms • Amplitude: >6.3 mV • Side-to-side difference: <50% • Conduction velocity: >44 m/s
AH, abductor hallucis.			
Source: From Buschbacher RM. Tibial nerve motor conduction to the abductor hallucis. *Am J Phys Med Rehabil.* 1999;78(6 suppl):S15–S20. PubMed PMID: 10573092.			

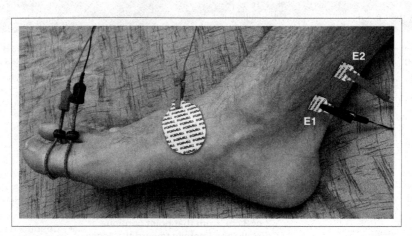

FIGURE 23.2 Tibial sensory nerve conduction studies medial plantar branch setup. E1 (black): Placement is posterior to and slightly proximal from the medial malleolus. E2 (gray): Placement is 4 cm proximal to E1. Ring electrodes placed on the great toe with cathode proximal and anode distal.

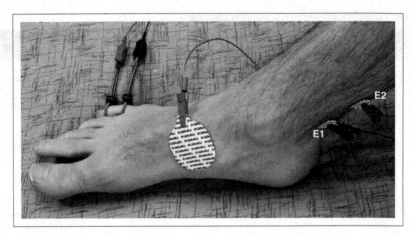

FIGURE 23.3 Tibial sensory nerve conduction studies lateral plantar branch setup. E1 (black): Placement is posterior to and slightly proximal from the medial malleolus. E2 (gray): Placement is 4 cm proximal to E1. Ring electrodes placed on the little toe with cathode proximal and anode distal.

TABLE 23.7 Tibial Mixed-Nerve Conduction Studies

Name	Lead Placement	Stimulation Site	Normal Values
Medial plantar mixed	• E1: Posterior to and slightly proximal from the medial malleolus; positioned just proximal to the flexor retinaculum • E2: 4 cm proximal to E1	A total of 14 cm distal to E1; first measure from E1 in a straight line to the sole of the foot inferior to the navicular prominence, likely to be 7 or 8 cm; from that point continue distally along the medial foot between the 1st and 2nd rays and place the cathode a total distance of 14 cm distal from E1	• Distal onset latency: ≤3.7 ms • Amplitude: ≥ 3 µV • Conduction velocity: >45 m/s
Lateral plantar mixed	• E1 and E2 placed same as described for medial plantar nerve	A total of 14 cm distal to E1; first measure from E1 in a straight line to the sole of the foot inferior to the navicular prominence, likely to be 7 or 8 cm; from that point continue distally and laterally toward the space between the 4th and 5th and place the cathode a total distance of 14 cm distal from E1	• Distal onset latency: ≤3.7 ms • Amplitude: ≥ 3 µV • Conduction velocity: > 45 m/s

Source: From Preston DC, Shapiro BE. Routine lower extremity nerve conduction techniques. In: *Electromyography and Neuromuscular Disorders: Clinical–Electrophysiologic Correlations.* 3rd ed. New York, NY: Elsevier Saunders; 2013:115–124.

TABLE 23.8 Delayed Responses

Name	Lead Placement	Stimulation Site	Normal Values
• Tibial F-wave	• E1: Over muscle belly of abductor hallucis 1 cm inferior and 1 cm proximal to the navicular prominence • E2: Placed more distally, over the metatarsophalangeal of the great toe	• Ankle: Posterior to the medial malleolus, 8 cm proximal from E1; catheter proximal, anode distal • Repetitive study, perform at least 10 recorded stimulations	• Minimal F-latency: ≤56 ms
• H-reflex	• E1: On posterior calf, halfway between the popliteal crease and the calcaneus, where the gastrocnemius and soleus join • E2: Over the Achilles tendon	• Over the tibial nerve in the midline of the popliteal fossa; cathode proximal and anode distal • Repetitive study, perform at least 10 recorded stimulations	• Minimal H-latency: ≤34 ms

Source: From Preston DC, Shapiro BE. Routine lower extremity nerve conduction techniques. In: *Electromyography and Neuromuscular Disorders: Clinical–Electrophysiologic Correlations.* 3rd ed. New York, NY: Elsevier Saunders; 2013:115–124.

TRADE SECRETS

- Tibial motor study can also be performed to the abductor digiti quinti; this tests the lateral plantar nerve terminal branch.
- The medial calcaneal branch may diverge from the main tibial nerve proximal to the tarsal tunnel, in which case tarsal tunnel syndrome would not involve the heel area.
- Tarsal tunnel syndrome is likely a rare clinical entity. One role for electrodiagnostic (EDX) studies is to evaluate for possible alternative diagnosis such as proximal tibial neuropathy, sciatic neuropathy, lumbosacral radiculopathy, or early peripheral polyneuropathy.
- A distal tibial lesion (e.g., the tarsal tunnel) may need to be differentiated from an S1 radiculopathy.
- A more proximal tibial nerve lesion may need to be differentiated from an L5 radiculopathy.
- Lower limb nerve injuries due to sports may involve the fibular (peroneal) or tibial nerves, with soccer-related injuries being a common causative factor in injuries to these nerves (1).
- In tarsal tunnel syndrome, sensory NCS are more likely to be abnormal than motor NCS (3).
- Sensory NCS abnormalities in tarsal tunnel may involve either or both of the distal branches in the foot, the medial, and lateral plantar nerves.

- Care must be taken when interpreting absent distal sensory NCS in older patients, as age-related absence of sensory potentials may be common in asymptomatic elderly individuals.
- Recent efforts have included high-resolution musculoskeletal ultrasound as an adjunctive modality in conjunction with EDX to provide objective data to support a clinical diagnosis. Much like in the median nerve at the carpal tunnel, distal tibial nerve pathology can be supported by the presence of local nerve swelling and an increased cross-sectional area on short axis ultrasound images. Diabetic patients with peripheral polyneuropathy were demonstrated to have a tibial nerve cross-sectional area 3 cm proximal to the medial malleolus of 22 mm^2 compared with 12 mm^2 for healthy, nondiabetic controls (4).

ADDITIONAL READINGS

Buschbacher RM. Reference values for peroneal nerve motor conduction to the tibialis anterior and for peroneal vs. tibial latencies. *Am J Phys Med Rehabil*. 2003;82(4):296–301. PubMed PMID: 12649656.

De Ruiter GC, Torchia ME, Amrami KK, Spinner RJ. Neurovascular compression following isolated popliteus muscle rupture: a case report. *J Surg Orthop Adv*. 2005;14(3):129–132. PubMed PMID: 16216180.

Lee HJ, DeLisa JA. *Manual of Nerve Conduction Study and Surface Anatomy for Needle Electromyography*. 4th ed. Philadelphia, PA: Lippincott Williams & Wilkins; 2005:80–86.

Mabin D. Distal nerve compression of the leg. Clinical and electrophysiologic study [in French]. *Neurophysiol Clin*. 1997;27(1):9–24. PubMed PMID: 9206760.

McCrory P, Bell S, Bradshaw C. Nerve entrapments of the lower leg, ankle and foot in sport. *Sports Med*. 2002;32(6):371–391. PubMed PMID: 11980501.

Peterson A, Kincaid JC. Rehabilitation of patients with neuropathies. In: Braddom RL, ed. *Physical Medicine and Rehabilitation*. 3rd ed. Philadelphia, PA: Saunders Elsevier; 2007:1086.

Preston DC, Shapiro BE. Tarsal tunnel syndrome. In: *Electromyography and Neuromuscular Disorders: Clinical–Electrophysiologic Correlations*. 3rd ed. New York, NY: Elsevier Saunders; 2013:115–124.

Saeed MA, Gatens PF. Compound nerve action potentials in the medial and lateral plantar nerves through the tarsal tunnel. *Arch Phys Med Rehabil*. 1982;63:304–307. PubMed PMID: 7092529.

REFERENCES

1. Kouyoumdijian JA. Peripheral nerve injuries: a retrospective survey of 456 cases. *Muscle Nerve*. 2006;34(6):785–788. doi:10.1002/mus.20624
2. Lau JT, Stavrou P. Posterior tibial nerve–primary. *Foot Ankle Clin*. 2004;9(2):271–285. doi:10.1016/j.fcl.2003.12.002
3. Patel AT, Gaines K, Malamut R, Park TA, Toro DR, Holland N; American Association of Neuromuscular and Electrodiagnostic Medicine. Usefulness of electrodiagnostic techniques in the evaluation of suspected tarsal tunnel syndrome: an evidence-based review. *Muscle Nerve*. 2005;32(2):236–240. doi:10.1002/mus.20393
4. Kunwarpal S, Kamlesh G, Sukhdeep K. High resolution ultrasonography of the tibial nerve in diabetic peripheral neuropathy. *J Ultrason*. 2017;17:246–252. doi:10.15557/JoU.2017.0036

Femoral Neuropathy

Dan Cushman

INTRODUCTION

Femoral nerve injuries are uncommon, and thus easily missed. The femoral nerve innervates the hip flexors and knee extensors, which are key muscle groups in ambulation. The saphenous nerve is a distal extension of the femoral nerve.

The most common causes for femoral nerve injury are iatrogenic from surgery, particularly abdominal and pelvic, related to lithotomy positioning or compression from retractors (1,2). Other possible causes affecting all or part of the femoral nerve include:

- Hematoma formation along iliopsoas due to anticoagulation
- Hip arthroplasties due to thermal injury, entrapment, compression
- Complications of femoral line placement, balloon angioplasty
- Saphenous nerve injury during graft harvesting of saphenous vein for bypass surgery
- Tumor or mass lesion
- Diabetes mellitus typically in the setting of diabetic amyotrophy
- Renal transplantation associated with steal phenomenon
- Infection or retroperitoneal abscess formation
- Bullet or stab wounds to the groin
- Spine surgery
- Urological procedures
- Knee surgery can injure the infrapatellar branch of the saphenous nerve, which supplies sensation to the inferomedial aspect of the knee

> **Clinical Pearls**
> - The saphenous nerve is a pure sensory branch of the femoral nerve. It may be difficult to locate with nerve conduction, so a contralateral examination can be helpful.
> - Keep in mind that the psoas muscle is innervated directly by the ventral rami of L1, L2, and L3, so there may be preservation of some hip flexion in a femoral nerve lesion.

CLINICAL PRESENTATION

History of present illness and physical examination are important components in electrodiagnostic assessment as they help the examiner to localize the lesion.

- Knee buckling possibly associated with loss of balance or falls
- Difficulty lifting leg (e.g., climbing stairs, getting out of car, getting out of chair)
- Dragging the leg during ambulation
- Numbness or paresthesias in the sensory distribution of the femoral nerve, which may involve the anteromedial thigh or medial aspect of lower leg and foot
- Pain in the anterior thigh and leg
- Physical examination may demonstrate deficits noted as follows; however, it is useful to compare the affected side with the unaffected side; in addition, the hip flexors and knee extensors are strong stabilizers and may need to be placed at a mechanical disadvantage in order to appreciate subtle weakness (3)
  - Physical examination should include testing of the hip adductors, which are also innervated by the L2–4 nerve roots, but a different peripheral nerve, the obturator nerve; this will help distinguish a femoral lesion from a lumbar plexopathy
- Atrophy of the quadriceps muscles
- Weakness on manual muscle testing of the iliacus or quadriceps muscles
- Diminished or absent reflexes at the knee
- Impaired or absent sensation in the sensory distribution of the femoral/saphenous nerve

Clinical Pearl
- Certain areas of the thigh are not innervated by the femoral cutaneous branches. The proximal medial thigh is supplied by the obturator nerve and sensation on the lateral aspect via the lateral femoral cutaneous nerve.

Clinical Pearls
- Physical examination should also include testing of hip adductors, which also receive contributions from L2–L4 nerve roots, but are innervated by a different peripheral nerve, the obturator nerve.
- Presence or absence of weakness in this muscle group may help to differentiate between a femoral lesion versus a plexopathy.

ANATOMY

- *Inguinal ligament:* A fibrous band that runs from the anterior superior iliac spine to pubic tubercle; a potential site for femoral nerve compression when the hip is flexed and externally rotated
- *Femoral triangle (Scarpa triangle):* A triangular space located in the anterior thigh; main contents are the femoral vessels, lymphatics, and the femoral nerve, which is located most laterally; boundaries of the femoral triangle include:
  - *Superior:* Inguinal ligament
  - *Medial:* Medial aspect of adductor longus muscle
  - *Lateral:* Lateral aspect of sartorius muscle
  - *Floor:* Adductor longus, pectineus, and iliopsoas
- *Hunter canal:* Also referred to as *adductor canal* or *subsartorial canal*, it is a fascial tunnel deep in the sartorius muscle along the anteromedial thigh; a potential site for entrapment of the saphenous nerve

Clinical Pearl
- Knee trauma or surgery can result in medial side knee pain related to injury of the infrapatellar branch of the saphenous nerve.

ELECTRODIAGNOSTIC APPROACH

- Nerve conduction study (NCS) can be quite uncomfortable due to nerve depth.
- Notes regarding the saphenous nerve (Tables 24.1–24.5):
  - It can be very challenging in general to obtain saphenous nerve conduction, so it is essential to perform side-to-side comparisons before considering the study abnormal.
  - There are two approaches to a saphenous nerve study: distal and proximal. The distal approach is described here. There is a proximal method, which can be more difficult in obese patients, that is described in detail by Buschbacher (4).
  - The saphenous nerve is a purely sensory continuation of the femoral nerve. An abnormal NCS, when compared with a normal asymptomatic side, may suggest a lesion with axonal loss distal from the nerve root, such as lumbar plexus or femoral nerve, which is peripheral. If normal, then the lesion is likely proximal to the dorsal root ganglia indicating a radiculopathy (5).

TABLE 24.1 Suggested Sensory Nerve Conduction Studies for Femoral Neuropathy

Test	Active Electrode	Reference Electrode	Stimulation Site
Saphenous (distal technique)	• A 3-cm bar is used • E1 is placed proximal and slightly medial to the tibialis anterior tendon	E2 is placed slightly anterior to the highest prominence of the medial malleolus, between the malleolus and the tendon of the tibialis anterior	14 cm proximal to E1 deep to the medial border of the tibia
Sural	• A 3-cm bar is used • E2 is placed distal to E1	E1 is placed behind the lateral malleolus	14 cm proximal to E1 in the midline or slightly lateral to the midline of the posterior lower leg

E1, active electrode; E2, reference electrode.
Note: Ground electrode should be placed between the stimulating and recording electrodes.
Source: Adapted from Buschbacher RM, Prahlow ND. *Manual of Nerve Conduction Studies.* 2nd ed. New York: Demos Medical Publishing; 2006.

TABLE 24.2 Normal Values

	Peak Latency (ms)	Amplitude (mV)
Saphenous (distal technique)	2.3–4.6	1–24
Sural	2.8–4.6	3–69

Note: Peak latency values represent upper limit of control. Amplitude values represent peak to peak.
Source: From Buschbacher RM. Sural and saphenous 14-cm antidromic sensory nerve conduction studies. *Am J Phys Med Rehabil.* 2003;82(6):421–426. PubMed PMID: 12820783.

TABLE 24.3 Suggested Motor Nerve Conduction Studies for Femoral Neuropathy

Test	Active Electrode	Reference Electrode	Stimulation Site
Femoral nerve to quadriceps	E1 is placed over the center of the vastus medialis muscle	E2 is placed over the quadriceps tendon just proximal to the patella	• Inferior to the inguinal ligament and lateral to the femoral artery
Tibial nerve to abductor hallucis	E1: 1 cm proximal and inferior to the navicular prominence	E2: Over the metatarsophalangeal joint of the great toe	• Medial ankle: Above and posterior to the medial malleolus at a point 9 cm proximal to E1 • Popliteal fossa: Midposterior knee over the popliteal pulse

(continued)

TABLE 24.3 Suggested Motor Nerve Conduction Studies for Femoral Neuropathy (*continued*)

Test	Active Electrode	Reference Electrode	Stimulation Site
Fibular nerve to extensor digitorum brevis	E1 is placed over the midpoint of the extensor digitorum brevis muscle on the dorsum of the foot	E2 is placed slightly distal to the 5th metatarsophalangeal joint	• Ankle: 8 cm proximal to E1, slightly lateral to the tibialis anterior tendon • Fibular head: Slightly posterior and inferior to the fibular head • Popliteal fossa: Approximately 10 cm proximal from the stimulation point at the fibular head and medial to the biceps femoris

E1, recording electrode; E2, reference electrode.

Source: Adapted from Buschbacher RM, Prahlow ND. *Manual of Nerve Conduction Studies.* 2nd ed. New York, NY: Demos Medical Publishing; 2006.

TABLE 24.4 Normal Values

	Onset Latency (ms)	Amplitude (mV)
Femoral nerve to rectus femoris (below inguinal ligament)	5.5–7.5	0.2–11.0
Tibial nerve to abductor hallucis	3.2–7.4	1.0–26.6
Fibular nerve extensor digitorum brevis	3.1–6.9	0.4–13.8

Note: Onset latency values represent upper limit of normal. Amplitude values represent peak to peak.

Source: Adapted from Buschbacher RM, Prahlow ND. *Manual of Nerve Conduction Studies.* 2nd ed. New York, NY: Demos Medical Publishing; 2006.

TABLE 24.5 Suggested Electromyographic Studies for Femoral Neuropathy

Motor	Needle Placement	Activation
Iliopsoas muscle	2 fingerbreadths lateral to the femoral pulse below the inguinal ligament	Flex the hip
Rectus femoris	Anterior thigh at the midpoint between the hip and the knee	Extend the knee and flex the hip while lifting the heel from bed
Adductor longus	Medial thigh 3–4 fingerbreadths distal to the pubis	Adduct the thigh
Tibialis anterior	Lateral to the tibial crest, two thirds the distance up from the ankle toward the knee	Dorsiflex the ankle

(*continued*)

TABLE 24.5 Suggested Electromyographic Studies for Femoral Neuropathy (*continued*)

Motor	Needle Placement	Activation
L2, L3, L4 paraspinals	• 2 fingerbreadths from the midline of the spine with needle directed medially • Advance to just touch the lamina then pull back slightly to ensure the needle	Assessed with patient at rest in side-lying position
Medial gastrocnemius	• Rostral medial posterior calf	Plantarflex the ankle

Source: From Preston DC, Shapiro BE. Femoral neuropathy. In: *Electromyography and Neuromuscular Disorders: Clinical–Electrophysiologic Correlations.* 2nd ed. Philadelphia, PA: Butterworth-Heinemann; 2005:184, 186, 189, 192, 358.

QUESTIONS

1. A possible site of entrapment for the saphenous nerve is:
   A. Hunter canal
   B. Inguinal ligament
   C. Posterior medial malleolus
   D. Extensor retinaculum of the ankle

2. An electromyography workup for femoral neuropathy should include:
   A. L2, L3, L4 paraspinals
   B. Rectus femoris
   C. Adductor longus
   D. All of the above

3. Which of these findings would be consistent with a femoral neuropathy?
   A. Abnormal compound muscle action potential of the adductor longus muscle
   B. Diminished sensation along the lateral surface of the thigh
   C. Prior history of abdominal or pelvic surgery
   D. Small bilateral saphenous nerve action potentials

4. A 40-year-old man on long-term anticoagulation therapy presents to your office with sudden-onset pain in the left anterior thigh with knee extension weakness that started 4 weeks ago. Nerve conduction studies show normal saphenous nerve responses bilaterally. What is the most likely diagnosis of the following options?
   A. Lumbosacral plexopathy
   B. L3 radiculopathy
   C. Saphenous mononeuropathy
   D. Femoral mononeuropathy

Answers to the questions are located in Chapter 35.

REFERENCES

1. Buschbacher RM. Sural and saphenous 14-cm antidromic sensory nerve conduction studies. *Am J Phys Med Rehabil*. 2003;82(6):421–426. PubMed PMID: 12820783.
2. Craig A. Entrapment neuropathies of the lower extremity. *PM & R*. 2013;5(5 suppl):S31–S40. doi:10.1016/j.pmrj.2013.03.029
3. Preston DC, Shapiro BE. Femoral neuropathy. In: *Electromyography and Neuromuscular Disorders: Clinical-Electrophysiologic Correlations*. 2nd ed. Philadelphia, PA: Butterworth-Heinemann; 2005:360–361.
4. Buschbacher RM, Prahlow, ND. *Manual of Nerve Conduction Studies*. New York, NY: Demos Medical Publishing LLC; 2006.
5. Dumitru D. Nerve conduction studies. In: *Electrodiagnostic Medicine*. 2nd ed. Philadelphia, PA: Hanley and Belfus; 2002:214–216.

25

Lumbosacral Radiculopathy

Nathan P. Olafsen and Daniel T. Probst

INTRODUCTION

- Radiculopathy, a disorder of the spinal nerve roots, is one of the most common diagnoses referred for electrodiagnostic (EDX) evaluation. It is important to remember that an EMG/nerve conduction study (NCS) is an extension of the history and physical examination. EDX studies should be ordered when the diagnosis remains unclear. EDX studies functionally assess the nerve, localize the lesion, and exclude other neurological causes of limb pain, sensory changes, and weakness.
  - EMG/NCS has a moderate degree of sensitivity (49%–86%) for assessing a radiculopathy. Reported specificity is variable, ranging from moderate to high (66%–100%) (1,2).
- Radiculopathy can be an axonal or demyelinating disorder affecting nerve fibers at the level of a single root or spinal nerve. The anterior (motor) root, posterior (sensory) root, or both may be affected. Pathology in the spinal nerve is less common.
  - In younger patients, radiculopathy is most commonly caused by a herniated disc. Radiculopathy in the elderly is most commonly caused by degenerative changes of the disc, uncovertebral joints, zygapophyseal joints, and/or ligamentous structures.

CLINICAL PRESENTATION

Radiculopathy commonly presents as pain and paresthesias along the dermatomal distribution of the affected nerve root. Weakness and reduced sensation may also be present in the myotomal and dermatomal distributions of the affected nerve root, and muscle stretch reflexes may be diminished. The differential diagnosis for lower extremity weakness and sensory changes is broad and includes, but is not limited to, radiculopathy, plexopathy, polyneuropathy, mononeuropathy, and nonneurologic musculoskeletal disorders. An understanding of spinal anatomy is essential to the performance and interpretation of EDX studies.

ANATOMY

There are 31 pairs of mixed spinal nerves attached along the length of the spinal cord: 8 cervical, 12 thoracic, 5 lumbar, 5 sacral, and 1 coccygeal. Each intervertebral foramen has an associated spinal nerve formed by the union of the ventral root and the dorsal root.

186 | Common Clinical Entities

The ventral root is composed of motor neurons whose cell bodies are located in the anterior horn of the spinal cord (Figure 25.1). The dorsal root is composed of bipolar, sensory neurons whose cell bodies are located in the dorsal root ganglion (DRG). The proximal end of the sensory nerve projects toward the spinal cord and the distal end projects away from the DRG toward the spinal nerve. After exiting the intervertebral foramen, each spinal nerve immediately splits into an anterior primary ramus and a posterior primary ramus. Each ramus is a mixed nerve with motor and sensory fibers. The anterior rami in the lumbosacral region join to form the lumbosacral plexus. The posterior rami innervate the paraspinal musculature and provide sensation over the back.

- As humans develop, the length of the vertebral column increases disproportionately compared to the length of the spinal cord. Therefore, the length of the spinal nerve roots increases progressively from the cervical spine downward.
- As a result of this disproportionate growth, the lumbar and sacral spinal roots must descend below the termination of the spinal cord, forming the cauda equina, to reach their respective intervertebral foramen. As these spinal roots descend through the lumbar spinal canal, they are at risk of compression throughout the course of their descent. Thus, depending on the size and location of a disc herniation, nerve roots from multiple lumbosacral levels could be compressed by a single disc (Figure 25.2).

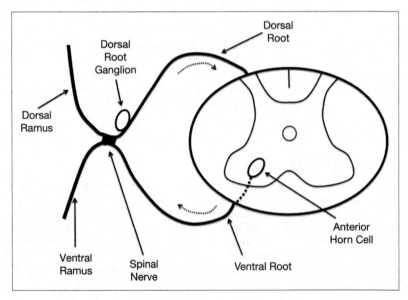

FIGURE 25.1 A cross-sectional image of the spinal cord demonstrating the anatomy of the anterior horn cell, ventral root, dorsal root ganglion, dorsal root, spinal nerve, and the ventral and dorsal rami.

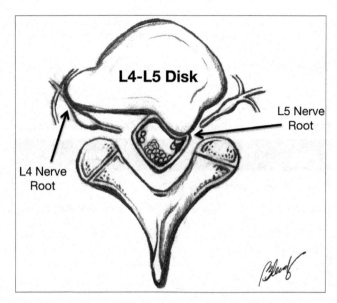

FIGURE 25.2 A posterolateral disc herniation, as pictured, can cause compression of the descending nerve root in the lateral recess of the spinal canal.

ELECTRODIAGNOSTIC APPROACH

In the setting of suspected lumbosacral radiculopathy, the goals of the EDX examination are to confirm evidence of a root involvement, to localize the pathology to either one or multiple root levels, and to exclude more distal or more generalized pathology. EDX cannot identify the exact cause of radiculopathy, but rather can only determine that axon loss has occurred (2). EDX is best used in a complementary role and to help confirm the diagnosis.

NERVE CONDUCTION STUDIES

NCS are usually normal in lumbar radiculopathies. However, sensory and motor NCS still need to be assessed as they help to exclude other disease processes included in the differential diagnosis.

- Sensory NCS:
  - Although a patient with radiculopathy may complain of numbness and tingling and may have sensory deficits on physical examination, sensory nerve action potentials (SNAPs) are typically normal in lumbosacral radiculopathy (3,4).
  - This concept is easy to remember by understanding the anatomy: Nerve root compression, in the setting of radiculopathy, usually occurs proximal to the DRG, where the sensory cell body is located. A SNAP is preserved as the sensory NCS only assesses the fibers distal to the DRG that are still in contact with the healthy cell body.

- The presence of a normal SNAP is useful in differentiating a radiculopathy from a more distal lesion (e.g., a plexopathy, mononeuropathy, or peripheral neuropathy), where the SNAP would be affected (1).
- Table 25.1 lists peripheral nerves commonly tested in sensory NCS and their respective nerve roots.

TABLE 25.1 Lower Limb Sensory Nerve Action Potential Studies

Nerve	Nerve Root
Lateral femoral cutaneous	L2 and L3
Saphenous	L4 and some L3
Superficial fibular	L5
Sural	S1

- Motor NCS:
  - Compound muscle action potentials (CMAPs) are usually normal in lumbosacral radiculopathies. However, abnormalities may be seen if a radiculopathy causes axonal loss. Again, this concept becomes clear with an understanding of spinal anatomy.
  - Unlike the sensory nerve cell bodies, which lie outside the central nervous system in the DRG and distal to a nerve root lesion, the cell body of the motor nerve lies in the anterior horn. Therefore, if the nerve root is compressed or irritated, the compression is distal to the cell body and Wallerian degeneration (axonal loss) may occur and then be detected with CMAP studies. If no axons are injured and only focal, proximal demyelination occurs, CMAPs will be normal as routine motor NCS only tests the distal portion of the nerves, which would still be myelinated normally.
  - It is important to remember that even in the setting of axonal loss, CMAPs may be normal in lumbosacral radiculopathy for the following reasons:
    - [ ] NCS are often normal in single root lesions as additional, unaffected roots supply the tested muscle masking potential abnormalities (4).
    - [ ] Root injury is often subtotal, with a small degree of axon loss that may be undetected on NCS (4).
  - Common muscles examined in routine lower limb motor NCS are the extensor digitorum brevis (fibular nerve and L5, S1) and abductor hallucis (tibial nerve and S1, S2).

LATE RESPONSES
- H-reflex:
  - The H-reflex is a true monosynaptic spinal reflex, which is obtained by stimulating the tibial nerve and recording over the gastrocsoleus muscle. The gastrocsoleus muscle is

the only muscle complex in the lower limb in which a relatively consistent H-reflex response can be obtained (4,5). As it is the electrical correlate of the ankle jerk reflex, it is useful in the evaluation of the S1 nerve root, but abnormality is not specific for radiculopathy and can also be seen in plexopathy, polyneuropathy, and peripheral neuropathy. As the H-reflex assesses the entire reflex arc, it becomes abnormal once nerve compression occurs, regardless of location.

- The H-reflex is assessed based on its latency or amplitude.
  - A normal H-reflex latency is less than 35 ms and is dependent on patient age, limb length, and height (1). A side-to-side onset latency difference of more than 1.0 to 1.5 ms or a latency that exceeds those predicted by a population nomogram is a criterion for diagnosing an S1 radiculopathy.
  - An abnormal H-amplitude is defined as 1 mV or less in patients younger than 60 years or a side-to-side amplitude difference of more than 50% on the symptomatic versus asymptomatic side (1). An absent or asymmetrically reduced H-amplitude can be found in 80% to 89% of surgically or myelographically confirmed cases of S1 radiculopathy (1).
- F-waves:
  - F-waves have poor sensitivity at detecting lumbosacral radiculopathies and add little to the diagnosis. Even when they are abnormal, their findings are often inconsequential because the needle examination will most likely be abnormal and more definitive. The sensitivity of F-waves is limited for the following reasons:
    - The sampled muscles are innervated by more than one nerve root. In a single-level radiculopathy, conduction through the normal roots can mask F-wave abnormalities.
    - F-waves assess the entire motor pathway and focal slowing over a short segment (as often seen in radiculopathy) may be diluted by normal conduction on the remainder of the pathway (1).
    - F-waves may miss abnormal fibers as they only assess motor fibers and only test 1% to 5% of the peripheral nerve fibers (6).

In summary, although often normal in radiculopathy, sensory and motor NCS should always be performed as their normality helps to rule out other diagnoses in the differential. The second component of the EDX examination, the needle EMG examination, is the most useful component of the EDX examination for the diagnosis of radiculopathy.

ELECTROMYOGRAPHY

The needle EMG examination is the most useful diagnostic tool in radiculopathy. It is felt to be the most sensitive aspect of the EDX examination for radiculopathy, although the report sensitivity ranges from 49% to 86% (2). EMG is considered a more specific than sensitive test. The diagnosis of radiculopathy by EMG requires the identification of neurogenic abnormalities in two or more muscles that share the same nerve root innervation but have a different peripheral nerve supply. Not all muscles within a myotome need to be affected. It is important to remember that EMG evaluates only motor fibers. Thus, not all radiculopathies can be confirmed by EMG, such as those with motor root demyelination without axon injury or those only impacting the sensory nerve root.

TABLE 25.2 Example of a Lower Limb Screen

Muscle	Peripheral Nerve	Nerve Root Innervation
Vastus medialis	Femoral	L2, L3, L4
Tibialis anterior	Deep fibular	L4, L5
Tensor fasciae latae	Superior gluteal	L4, L5, S1
Peroneus longus	Superficial fibular	L5, S1
Medial gastrocnemius	Tibial	S1, S2
Lumbosacral paraspinal muscles		

- EMG approach:
  - One of the purposes of an EMG screen is to identify radiculopathy that can be confirmed by EMG. It is important to maximize the number of muscles included in the screen to be able to identify or exclude a radiculopathy that could be confirmed by EMG. When paraspinal muscles are included as a part of the radiculopathy screen, a screen of six muscles (five limb plus paraspinals), representing all lumbosacral nerve root levels, will identify 98% to 100% of lumbosacral radiculopathies (7). An example of this type of screen can be seen in Table 25.2.
  - If paraspinal muscles cannot be reliably included (see text that follows), a screening of eight distal muscles is necessary to identify approximately 90% of radiculopathies (7).
    - In either type of screen, whenever an abnormal muscle is encountered, additional muscles should be tested to determine the nature and location of pathology.
  - The specific muscles to sample when screening for radiculopathy are at the discretion of the examiner. Some general recommendations are as follows (8):
    - Sample muscles within the same myotome but innervated by different peripheral nerves to exclude a mononeuropathy.
    - Sample both proximal and distal muscles of the same myotome to exclude a distal-to-proximal pattern of abnormalities that may occur in a peripheral neuropathy.
    - Sample muscles innervated by myotomes above and below the suspected lesion level to exclude a more widespread or diffuse process.
  - In the majority of patients, paraspinal muscles should be sampled to help differentiate radiculopathy from plexopathy.
    - Caution should be exercised when diagnosing a radiculopathy on EMG based solely on paraspinal muscle abnormalities, especially in those over 40 years old. It is important to remember that paraspinal spontaneous activity is not pathognomonic of radiculopathy and may also be seen in patients with spinal cancers, amyotrophic lateral sclerosis, and following lumbar puncture.

Furthermore, in patients who have undergone lumbar posterior spinal surgery, the sampling of paraspinal muscles should be avoided as abnormalities may be related to damage of the posterior primary rami during surgery.
- Time course of EMG findings:
  - When radiculopathy causes axonal loss, the time course of the examination is important in order to interpret the findings properly. Within 3 days of injury, the only finding on EMG will be decreased recruitment due to the compression of axons.
  - After the axonal injury has been present for 1 to 2 weeks, fibrillation potentials and positive sharp waves may be observed in the paraspinal muscles. Fibrillation potentials and positive sharp waves then progress in a proximal-to-distal pattern appearing in the proximal limb muscles 2 to 3 weeks postinjury and in the distal limb muscles 3 to 4 weeks postinjury.
  - After 2 to 3 months, fibrillations and sharp waves become progressively smaller and begin to disappear as denervation decreases. As reinnervation and collateral sprouting begin, motor unit action potentials become large and polyphasic. Complex, repetitive discharges may also be seen in the more chronic radicular lesion. Using these general temporal guidelines, one can determine the proper time to perform an EMG postinjury, and based on the EMG results, estimate the chronicity of the lesion.

Clinical Pearls

- SNAPs are usually normal in radiculopathy despite the presence of clinical sensory abnormalities.
- A radiculopathy screen should sample six muscles if paraspinal muscles are included. If paraspinal muscles are not included, eight distal limb muscles should be screened.
- Use caution when diagnosing radiculopathy based only on abnormal paraspinal muscle potentials.
- Based on the EMG findings, one can estimate the time course of a lesion.

SUMMARY

The EDX evaluation of lumbosacral radiculopathy is an extension of the history and physical examination. It is a specific, but not robustly sensitive, test that should be performed when the diagnosis is unclear, to help delineate the level of nerve root pathology, and to exclude more distal or more generalized pathology. NCSs are usually normal in lumbosacral radiculopathies. The needle EMG is most helpful in localizing the pathology and determining the chronicity of the lesion.

QUESTIONS

1. When should an EMG be performed to assess for a lumbosacral radiculopathy?
   A. When an orthopedic physician consults you for one.
   B. When the diagnosis remains unclear after a proper history and physical and imaging studies.
   C. If a patient has a herniated disc at L4–5 on magnetic resonance imaging.
   D. Following a referral from the emergency department the day of an acute lifting injury producing pain in the lower back and numbness and tingling in the L5 distribution.

2. Which of the following statements explains why sensory nerve action potentials (SNAPs) are usually normal in lumbosacral radiculopathies?
   A. Nerve root compression in radiculopathy usually occurs proximal to the sensory dorsal root ganglion (DRG). The region of the nerve examined with the SNAP techniques assesses only the fibers distal to the DRG that are still in contact with the healthy cell body.
   B. Nerve root compression in radiculopathy usually occurs distal to the sensory DRG. The region of the nerve examined with the SNAP techniques assesses only the fibers distal to the DRG that are still in contact with the healthy cell body.
   C. Nerve root compression is distal to the anterior horn cell of the spinal cord.
   D. Lumbar radiculopathies usually result in Wallerian degeneration of the sensory axon distally.

3. How many muscles should be sampled on EMG for a lumbosacral radiculopathy screen?
   A. Three muscles plus three different areas of the paraspinal muscles
   B. Five limb muscles plus the paraspinal muscles
   C. Eight limb muscles if paraspinal muscles are not sampled
   D. B and C

REFERENCES

1. Katiriji B. Case 2 focal disorders. In: Katiriji B, ed. *Electromyography in Clinical Practice: A Case Study Approach*. St. Louis, MO: Mosby; 1998:13–27.
2. Dillingham TR. Evaluating the patient with suspected radiculopathy. *PM & R*. 2013;5(5):S41–S49. doi:10.1016/j.pmrj.2013.03.015
3. Dumitru D, Zwarts MJ. Radiculopathies. In: Dumitru D, Amato AA, Zwarts MJ, eds. *Electrodiagnostic Medicine*. 2nd ed. Philadelphia, PA: Hanley & Belfus; 2002:713–776.
4. Berger AR, Sharma K, Lopton RB. Comparison of motor conduction abnormalities in lumbosacral radiculopathy and axonal polyneuropathy. *Muscle Nerve*. 1999;22:1053–1057. PubMed PMID: 10417786.

Answers to the questions are located in Chapter 35.

5. Braddom RI, Johnson EW. Standardization of H-reflex and diagnostic use in S1 radiculopathy. *Arch Phys Med Rehabil*. 1974;55:161–166. PubMed PMID: 4823067.
6. Aminoff MJ, Goodin DS, Parry GJ, et al. Electrophysiologic evaluation of lumbosacral radiculopathies: Electromyography, late response, and somatosensory evoked potentials. *Neurology*. 1985;35:1514–1518. PubMed PMID: 2993952.
7. Dillingham TR. Electrodiagnostic medicine II: clinical evaluation and findings. In: Braddom RL, Buschbacher RM, Chan L, et al, eds. *Physical Medicine & Rehabilitation*. 3rd ed. Philadelphia, PA: Elsevier Inc; 2007:201–226.
8. Preston D, Shapiro B. Late responses. In: *Electromyography and Neuromuscular Disorders*. 2nd ed. Philadelphia, PA: Elsevier Science; 2005:459–478.

Cervical Radiculopathy

Ryan Doyel and Monica E. Rho

INTRODUCTION

Cervical radiculopathy results from a disruption of the nerve roots from the cervical spine. It occurs much less frequently than lumbar radiculopathy (1). Electrodiagnostic studies are a useful tool to supplement history and physical examination in the diagnosis of a cervical radiculopathy.

CLINICAL PRESENTATION

Causes

- Herniated nucleus pulposus
- Degenerative spondylosis, often with ligament hypertrophy
- Spondylolisthesis
- Tumor or mass (including granulomatous tissue, abscess, cyst)
- Infection

Classic Clinical Symptoms

- Pain and paresthesias along a dermatomal distribution of a specific cervical nerve root
- Weakness following the myotomal distribution of a specific cervical nerve root
- Abnormal muscle stretch reflexes (MSR), if the level of radiculopathy correlates with a particular myotomal distribution
  - Biceps and brachioradialis MSR: C5 and C6
  - Triceps MSR: C7 mainly, but does have some C6 and C8 contributions
- Symptom provocation with upper limb neural tension testing (high sensitivity, low specificity) (2)

Given dermatomal overlap, it is unusual to see a severe sensory disturbance with a cervical monoradiculopathy. Also, given the fact that most muscles are innervated by multiple myotomes and nerve roots, it is uncommon to have absent strength in one muscle following a monoradiculopathy.

ANATOMY OF THE CERVICAL SPINE

- Six cervical discs (no disc between C1 and C2)
- Seven vertebrae (C1–C7)
- Eight pairs of spinal nerves (C1–C8)

SPINAL NERVES

- Cervical spinal nerves exit the spinal column above the level of their similarly numbered cervical vertebrae (C8 exits above T1 vertebra) (Figures 26.1 and 26.2)
- Are composed of the ventral root (motor fibers) whose cell body is in the anterior horn of the spinal cord, and the dorsal root (sensory fibers) whose cell body is outside the spinal cord in the dorsal root ganglion
- Consist of both sensory and motor fibers
- Divide into the ventral ramus (anterior primary ramus) and the dorsal ramus (posterior primary ramus) at the intervertebral foramen; both rami are considered to be mixed nerves with motor and sensory fibers running within them
- The dorsal rami innervate the paraspinal muscles and the skin of the back
- The ventral rami continue distally to form a plexus; the upper cervical ventral rami (C1–C4) form the cervical plexus, which extends to innervate the scalene and strap neck muscles as well as the skin of the neck; the lower cervical ventral rami (C5–C8), along with the T1 ventral ramus, form the brachial plexus, which extends to innervate the muscles and skin of the upper limb (3)

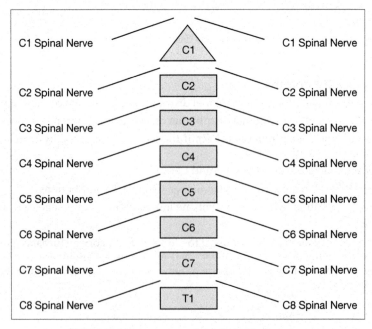

FIGURE 26.1 Orientation of cervical spinal nerves.

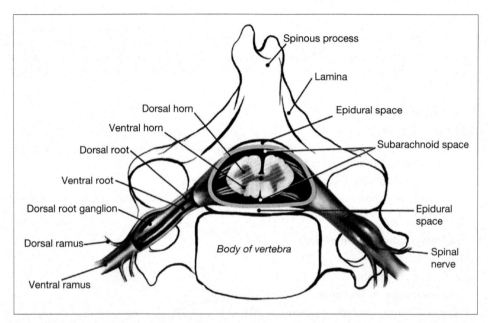

FIGURE 26.2 Cervical spine cross-section.
Source: From Cuccurullo SJ. *Physical Medicine and Rehabilitation Board Review.* 2nd ed. New York, NY: Demos Medical Publishing; 2010:387.

ELECTRODIAGNOSTIC APPROACH

The optimal evaluation of a patient with suspected radiculopathy is at least one motor and one sensory nerve conduction study (NCS) in the involved limb (4). The utility of the NCS in a cervical radiculopathy examination is to exclude polyneuropathy or plexopathy.

Motor Nerve Conduction Study

The motor nerve conduction study is expected to be normal if the injury is purely demyelinating, incomplete, or reinnervation has already occurred. Otherwise, there will be reduced compound muscle action potential amplitude in the case of severe disease.

Sensory Nerve Conduction Study

The sensory nerve conduction study is expected to be normal because in radiculopathy the lesion is usually proximal to the dorsal root ganglion.

Late Responses

F-Waves

- Poor sensitivity and specificity for cervical radiculopathy
- Tests only 1% to 5% of fibers and can miss abnormal fibers
- Muscles have multiple root innervations and F-wave latency may reflect only the healthy fibers

H-Reflex
- Not necessary in cervical radiculopathy examination
- Very rarely done in upper limbs, with recording over the flexor carpi radialis muscle and stimulating the median nerve to evaluate for a C6–7 radiculopathy; prolonged latency is most often due to C7 radiculopathy (5).

Electromyography

Diagnostic Criteria
- Electromyographic abnormalities in two or more muscles innervated by the same nerve root and different peripheral nerves (6)
- Muscles innervated by adjacent nerve roots are normal
- Other conditions are excluded (e.g., mononeuropathy, polyneuropathy, or brachial plexopathy)

Electromyography Abnormalities
- Positive sharp waves
- Fibrillation potentials
- Complex repetitive discharges
- Polyphasic motor unit action potentials (MUAP)
- High-amplitude, long-duration MUAP
- Reduced recruitment

Note: The presence of pain and paresthesias in a classic dermatomal distribution without electrodiagnostic abnormality is suggestive of nerve irritation without damage and is termed *radiculitis* rather than *radiculopathy*.

Muscle Testing
An optimal cervical radiculopathy screen includes five upper limb muscles plus the cervical paraspinals. If cervical paraspinal muscles cannot be tested (as is the case with a history of cervical spinal operative repair), testing eight upper limb muscles is recommended (7). If a muscle is found to be abnormal, more muscles should be tested based on the site of the suspected lesion. Table 26.1 refers to a sample screen.

TABLE 26.1 Sample Electromyography Muscle Screen for a Cervical Radiculopathy

Muscle	Nerve Root Level	Peripheral Nerve
Deltoid	C5–C6	Axillary
Biceps	C5–C6	Musculocutaneous
Pronator teres	C6–C7	Median
Triceps	C7–C8	Radial
First dorsal interosseous	C8–T1	Ulnar
Cervical paraspinals	C1–C8	Cervical dorsal rami

QUESTIONS

1. A 28-year-old male was involved in a high-speed motor vehicle collision with airbag deployment. You see him in your office 3 weeks after the collision with persistent pain in his neck radiating down his right shoulder to the dorsal side of his forearm, and progressive weakness of right elbow extension, wrist extension, and forearm pronation. Muscle stretch reflexes are 2+ at the left triceps, bilateral biceps, and brachioradialis muscles and 0 at the right triceps muscle. MRI of the cervical spine demonstrates a large disc herniation. What best represents the location of the disc herniation?
   A. C6–7 disc herniation impinging on the C7 spinal nerve
   B. C6–7 disc herniation impinging on the C6 spinal nerve
   C. C7–8 disc herniation impinging on the C7 spinal nerve
   D. C7–8 disc herniation impinging on the C8 spinal nerve

2. A 38-year-old female came for electrodiagnostic evaluation of numbness and tingling of her right hand, especially around the first three digits of her hand. Motor and sensory nerve conduction studies (NCS) of the median and radial nerves are normal. EMG demonstrates normal deltoids, biceps, and abductor pollicis brevis muscles on the right and spontaneous activity in the triceps, extensor carpi radialis, and extensor carpi ulnaris muscles on the right. Which of the following is true?
   A. This is a right C7 radiculopathy
   B. This is a right radial nerve mononeuropathy
   C. This study is inconclusive and no further testing can be completed
   D. This study is inconclusive and the right pronator teres should be tested by EMG

3. A 31-year-old male football player presents for electrodiagnostic evaluation of right neck and shoulder pain for 5 weeks. Symptoms have progressed since completion of a game during which he endured prolonged time underneath multiple players in a scrum for a loose ball. He was in a prone position, with neck held in full left lateral flexion during the time of impact. Physical examination is notable for shoulder abduction weakness and tightness of posterior neck musculature bilaterally. Motor and sensory NCS of median, ulnar, and radial nerves are normal. EMG demonstrates increased spontaneous activity in deltoid and biceps, with normal activity in triceps, flexor carpi radialis, and first dorsal interosseous. What further electrodiagnostic testing is most useful in the etiologic workup?
   A. EMG of middle cervical paraspinal muscles
   B. EMG of anconeus
   C. Sensory NCS of lateral antebrachial cutaneous nerve
   D. No further testing is necessary to determine etiology

Answers to the questions are located in Chapter 35.

4. A 24-year-old female came for electrodiagnostic testing after a motor vehicle collision 2 months ago. She has had persistent right arm pain and weakness since that collision. Her sensory and motor NCS of the median nerve were normal. Her electromyographic testing is below.

Muscles	Positive Sharp Waves	Fibrillations
Deltoid	None	None
Biceps	2+	1+
Triceps	None	None
Extensor carpi radialis	2+	1+
Pronator teres	1+	1+
Extensor indicis proprius	None	None
Abductor pollicis brevis	None	None
Middle cervical paraspinals	2+	1+

Which location of injury would best explain the EMG findings?
A. C6 ventral ramus
B. C6 ventral root
C. C6 dorsal ramus
D. C6 dorsal root

5. A 53-year-old female with a history of rheumatoid arthritis and prior C1–C2 posterior spinal arthrodesis is referred by a neurosurgeon for electrodiagnostic evaluation of left shoulder flexion and elbow flexion weakness amid neck pain. Motor and sensory NCS of the median and ulnar nerves are normal. Electromyographic screen reveals the following:

Muscles	Positive Sharp Waves	Fibrillations
Deltoid	2+	1+
Biceps	2+	None
Triceps	None	None
Pronator teres	None	None
First dorsal interosseous	None	None

What further electrodiagnostic testing should be completed to determine the specific level of radicular injury?
A. NCS of radial nerve with recording over extensor indicis proprius
B. EMG of middle cervical paraspinals
C. EMG of rhomboids
D. No further testing is necessary to determine a specific level of lesion

REFERENCES

1. Ahlgren BD, Garfin SR. Cervical radiculopathy. *Orthop Clin North Am.* 1996;27:253–262. PubMed PMID: 8614578.
2. Rubinstein SM, Pool JJM, van Tulder MW, et al. A systematic review of the diagnostic accuracy of provocative tests of the neck for diagnosing cervical radiculopathy. *Eur Spine J.* 2007;16(3):307–319. doi:10.1007/s00586-006-0225-6
3. Jenkins DB. *Hollinshead's Functional Anatomy of the Limbs and Back.* Philadelphia, PA: Saunders; 2002:251–253.
4. American Association of Electrodiagnostic Medicine. Guidelines in electrodiagnostic medicine. *Muscle Nerve.* 1999;(suppl 8):S53–S69. PMID 16921627.
5. Zheng C, Zhu Y, Lv F, et al. Abnormal flexor carpi radialis H-reflex as a specific indicator of C7 as compared with C6 radiculopathy. *J Clin Neurophysiol.* 2014;31(6):529–534. doi:10.1097/WNP.0000000000000104.
6. Wilbourn AJ, Aminoff MJ. AAEM mini-monograph 32: the electrodiagnostic examination in patients with radiculopathies. *Muscle Nerve.* 1998;21:1612–1631. PubMed PMID: 9843062.
7. Dillingham TR, Lauder TD, Andary M, et al. Identification of cervical radiculopathies: optimizing the electromyographic screen. *Am J Phys Med Rehabil.* 2001;80:84–91. PubMed PMID: 11212017.

27

Facial Nerve and Blink Studies

Kevin Carneiro and William Filer

INTRODUCTION
- Facial neuropathy is the most common cranial neuropathy
- Most commonly unilateral (1)

CLINICAL PRESENTATION
- Diabetes and pregnancy are predisposing conditions
  - May also be associated with infection, such as herpes zoster (Ramsay Hunt syndrome) or Lyme disease
- Usually presents as paresis or paralysis of upper and lower facial muscles ipsilateral to the facial nerve lesion

ANATOMY
Upper Motor Neuron
- In the face, originate from the primary motor cortex and control contralateral lower motor neurons
- Upper motor neuron lesions spare the upper face (Figure 27.1)

Lower Motor Neuron
- Motor root:
  - From facial nucleus in caudal lateral pons
  - Fibers make loop around nucleus of cranial nerve (CN) VI → cerebellopontine cistern → external acoustic meatus

- Sensory root (nervus intermedius):
  - Consists of parasympathetic, visceral sensory, and general somatosensory fibers
    - They arise from superior salivary nucleus, nucleus solitarius, and spinal trigeminal nucleus, respectively
  - Separate from motor root between the brainstem and internal acoustic meatus

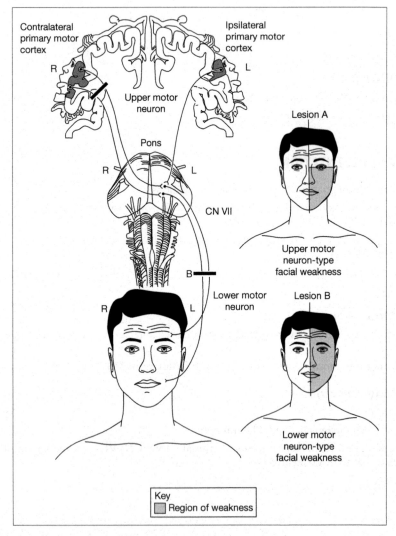

FIGURE 27.1 Upper motor neuron versus lower motor neuron weakness.

Source: With permission from Blumenfeld H. *Neuroanatomy Through Clinical Cases*. Sunderland, MA: Sinauer Associates Inc.; 2002:483.

- Facial nerve:
  - Travels in the internal auditory meatus → geniculate ganglion (cell bodies of general somatic and special visceral sensory that branch out here) → rest of nerve goes through facial canal → stylomastoid foramen → divides into branches (temporal, zygomatic, buccal, mandibular, and cervical)
  - Branchial motor → muscles of facial expression, posterior belly of digastric, stapedius, stylohyoid
  - Parasympathetic → soft palate, all salivary glands (except parotid) and lacrimal glands
  - Special visceral sensory → taste to the anterior $\frac{2}{3}$ of the tongue
  - Somatic sensory → small part of the external auditory meatus and skin of the ear

ELECTRODIAGNOSTIC APPROACH
Nerve Conduction Studies
Common approaches include facial motor studies and the blink reflex. The facial motor study assesses the peripheral efferent motor pathway of CN VII, whereas the blink reflex involves afferent conduction via CN V and efferent conduction along CN VII. The blink reflex is most useful when localization of the lesion is in question.

- Facial nerve motor conduction study (Figure 27.2):
  - *Active electrode (G1):* Nasalis muscle (lateral and 1 cm above the external nares)
  - *Reference electrode (G2):* Placed on the opposite nasalis muscle or on bridge of nose
  - *Stim site:* Below and anterior to the mastoid process
  - *Key points:*
    - Watch for and avoid direct stimulation of the masseter muscle, which would cause initial positivity
    - Distances from cathode to recording electrode must be equal
    - Alternative recording sites include orbicularis oculi and orbicularis oris muscles
    - Compound muscle action potential (CMAP) amplitude <10% of the contralateral side confers worse prognosis for spontaneous recovery (2), and it may be helpful to identify those who would benefit from early surgical decompression (3)
- Blink reflex (Figure 27.3):
  - *Active electrodes (G1):* Bilateral orbicularis oculi on inferior orbits
  - *Reference electrodes (G2):* Bilateral lateral canthus
  - *Stim site:* Supraorbital notch
  - *Key points:*
    - Recordings are made simultaneously on both sides
    - R_1 (early oligosynaptic ipsilateral response) and R_2 (late bilateral polysynaptic response)
    - R_1 afferent—V_1 to main sensory nucleus of CN V in pons
    - R_2 afferent—V_1 to spinal nucleus through polysynaptic pathway in pons and medulla
    - R_1 and R_2 efferent—CN VII motor

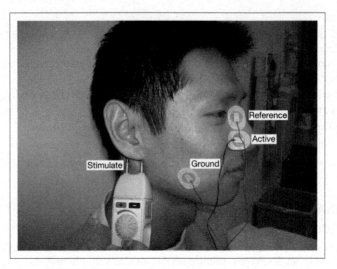

FIGURE 27.2 Facial nerve motor conduction study.

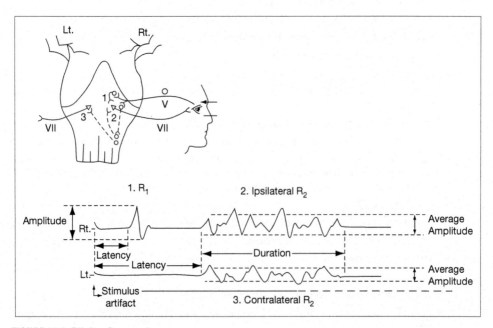

FIGURE 27.3 Blink reflex study.

Source: With permission from Kimura J. The blink reflex. In: *Electrodiagnosis in Diseases of Nerve and Muscle: Principles and Practice.* 3rd ed. New York, NY: Oxford University Press; 2001:409–438.

- Slowly increase current and R_2 will usually appear before R_1
- In facial neuropathy, the R_1 and R_2 responses will be abnormal ipsilaterally and normal contralaterally
- In trigeminal nerve lesions, ipsilateral R_1 and bilateral R_2 responses will be abnormal (Tables 27.1–27.3)

TABLE 27.1 Causes of Facial Neuropathy

Common Causes	Less Common Causes
• Bell's palsy (idiopathic) • Ramsay Hunt syndrome (herpes zoster virus)	• Fractures • Infections (middle ear, Lyme, mumps, human immunodeficiency virus, etc.) • Neoplasms (cerebellopontine angle tumors, lymphoma) • Multiple sclerosis • Inflammatory polyneuropathies (Guillain–Barré, Miller Fisher syndrome)

TABLE 27.2 Facial Nerve Motor Study Normal Values

Amplitude (mV)	Latency (ms)
≥1.0	≤4.2
Latency difference <0.6	

Source: From Preston DC. Detailed Nerve Conduction Studies. In: Preston DC, ed. *Electromyography and Nerve Conduction Disorders*. London, UK: Elsevier; 2016:97–114.

TABLE 27.3 Blink Reflex Study Normal Values

Response	Latency	Side-to-Side Latency Difference
R_1 (ipsateral)	≤13	≤1.2
R_2 (ipsilateral)	≤41	≤5
R_2 (contralateral)	≤44	≤7

Source: From Preston DC. Detailed Nerve Conduction Studies. In: Preston DC, ed. *Electromyography and Nerve Conduction Disorders*. London, UK: Elsevier; 2016:97–114.

Electromyography

Needle electromyography may be used to demonstrate motor activity and/or denervation in selected facial muscles. It does not require comparison to a normal contralateral side and thus may be helpful diagnostically when bilateral pathology is present. Muscles commonly sampled include frontalis, orbicularis oris, orbicularis oculi, and mentalis.

QUESTIONS

1. Where do you place the recording electrode when performing a facial motor nerve conduction study, stimulating anterior to the mastoid process?
   A. Over the ipsilateral orbicularis oculi muscle
   B. Over the contralateral orbicularis oculi muscle
   C. Over the ipsilateral nasalis muscle
   D. Over the contralateral nasalis muscle

2. During a teaching-rounds session, your attending physician presents to you an electrodiagnostic challenge. She states that you have performed a blink reflex study and have obtained the following information:
   - Stimulation of the left supraorbital notch produces a delayed R_1 with prolongation of bilateral R_2 responses.
   - Stimulation of the right supraorbital notch produces normal R_1 and bilateral R_2 responses.

   What clinical condition does this patient have?
   A. Left facial neuropathy
   B. Right facial neuropathy
   C. Left trigeminal neuropathy
   D. Left chorda tympani neuropathy

3. A 23-year-old man is sent to the electrophysiology laboratory for evaluation of left-sided facial droop. He undergoes a direct facial nerve motor study 1 week after he notices his symptoms. Amplitude is 0.5 mV compared with 2 mV on the contralateral side. Ipsilateral latency is 4.0 ms and latency difference is 0.6 ms. Which measurement can best be used to predict the prognosis?
   A. Amplitude
   B. Latency
   C. Latency difference
   D. It is too early to determine prognosis

Answers to the questions are located in Chapter 35.

4. Which of the following studies is most helpful in the early localization of an acute proximal lesion of the facial nerve?
   A. Facial motor nerve conduction study
   B. Blink reflex
   C. Needle electromyography of the frontalis muscle
   D. None of the above

ADDITIONAL READINGS

Byun H, Jang JY, Chung KW, et al. Value of electroneurography as a prognostic factor for recovery in acute severe inflammatory facial paralysis: a prospective study of Bell's palsy and Ramsay Hunt syndrome. *Laryngoscope.* 2013;123(10):2526–2532. doi:10.1002/lary.23988

Kennelly KD. Electrodiagnostic approach to cranial neuropathies. *Neurol Clin.* 2012;30(2):661–684. doi:10.1016/j.ncl.2011.12.014

Pearce J. Observations on the blink reflex. *Eur Neurol.* 2008;59:221–223. doi:10.1159/000114053

REFERENCES

1. Gilchrist J. Seventh cranial neuropathy. *Semin Neurol.* 2009;29(1):5–13. doi:10.1055/s-0028-1124018
2. May M, Blumenthal F, Klein SR. Acute Bell's palsy: prognostic value of evoked electromyography, maximal stimulation, and other electrical tests. *Am J Otol.* 1983;5:1–7. PubMed PMID: 6881304
3. Gantz BJ, Rubinstein JT, Gidley P, et al. Surgical management of Bell's palsy. *Laryngoscope.* 1999;109(8):1177–1188. doi:10.1097/00005537-199908000-00001

28

Repetitive Stimulation and Neuromuscular Junction Disorders

Trevor Gessel and Nassim Rad

INTRODUCTION
The use of repetitive stimulation (RS) techniques for assessment of disorders of neuromuscular transmission is an important skill for any electrodiagnostic (EDX) consultant in the evaluation of a patient with generalized weakness. The differential diagnosis for generalized weakness is broad and includes neuropathies, myopathies, motor neuron disease, and neuromuscular junction (NMJ) disorders.

CLINICAL PRESENTATION
- NMJ disorders typically present with generalized weakness and easy fatigability
  - Sensory complaints are not a usual part of the presentation of these conditions.
- Myasthenia gravis (MG):
  - Most common and well-defined NMJ disorder
  - Antibodies directed against the acetylcholine receptors on the *postsynaptic* membrane in the majority of cases
  - Involves the proximal muscles much more than the distal
  - Ptosis, dysarthria, and dysphagia can be a presenting complaint
- Lambert–Eaton myasthenic syndrome (LEMS):
  - Second most common NMJ disorder
  - Often associated with paraneoplastic conditions such as small cell carcinoma of the lung
  - Antibodies directed against the voltage-gated calcium channels in the *presynaptic* membrane.
  - Autoimmune complaints (i.e., dry mouth) may be present
  - Less likely to complain of ptosis, dysarthria, or dysphagia

- Botulism:
  - Usually an infantile or foodborne illness
  - Botulinum toxin cleaves SNARE (SNAP [sensory nerve action potential] receptor) complex proteins to prevent vesicles containing acetylcholine from docking with the *presynaptic* membrane
- Other causes of NMJ disorders:
  - Congenital myasthenic syndromes, poisonings (snake venom, black widow venom, organophosphates, insecticides), hypermagnesemia

ELECTRODIAGNOSTIC APPROACH
Nerve Conduction Studies
At least one sensory and one motor nerve in one upper and one lower limb should be tested to screen for generalized polyneuropathy and motor neuron disease. F-waves should generally be included when assessing a patient with generalized weakness.

> **Clinical Pearl**
> - Diffusely low compound muscle action potentials (CMAPs) should raise concern for LEMS.

Electromyography
At least one upper and one lower limb should be tested to assess for a neurogenic or myopathic source of weakness, sampling proximal and distal muscles.

Repetitive Stimulation
- Follow these steps in the order given (Tables 28.1–28.3):
  - Establish the supramaximal compound muscle action potentials (CMAP).
  - Perform slow (2–3 Hz) RS (train of 5–10) to assess for decrement. Repeat after a few minutes to ensure reproducibility.
  - Exercise the muscle for 10 seconds then reassess with slow RS to assess for postexercise facilitation. Repeat after a few minutes to ensure reproducibility.
  - Have the patient actively exercise the muscle maximally for 60 seconds, then assess with single supramaximal stimulations every 30 to 60 seconds for the next 4 to 6 minutes to evaluate for postexercise exhaustion.
  - Fast RS (20–30 Hz to produce exercise effect and 50 Hz for producing tetany) should only be used, if necessary, in patients who cannot provide voluntary muscle contraction, as fast RS is very painful.

> **Clinical Pearls**
> - *Movement Artifact:* Attention must be given to ensure that the recording electrodes remain stable during RS as even slight movement can produce artifactually abnormal results. The stimulator must also remain stable; otherwise, submaximal stimulation can potentially be delivered to some responses.
> - *Temperature:* There is decreased sensitivity for decremental response with cool limb temperatures. Temperature should be monitored during the evaluation and effort should be made to maintain skin temperature above 34°C during RS testing.

Single Fiber

Single-fiber EMG should be considered when RS testing is normal or equivocal and there remains a high suspicion for an NMJ disorder. It is highly sensitive in assessing for increased jitter or blocking, which suggests instability of the NMJ.

TABLE 28.1 Definitions

Common Terms Used in Repetitive Stimulation	Definition
Decrement	A reproducible decline in the amplitude and/or area of the CMAP of successive responses to repetitive nerve stimulation.
Increment	A reproducible increase in amplitude and/or area of successive CMAPs to repetitive nerve stimulation.
Jitter	Variability in interpotential interval between consecutive discharges of two muscle fiber action potentials belonging to the same motor unit, seen on single-fiber needle electromyography.
Postexercise exhaustion	A reduction in the safety factor of neuromuscular transmission after sustained activation at the neuromuscular junction. Usually identified as a more significant decremental response.
Postexercise facilitation	An increase in an electrically measured response to identical stimuli after sustained activation at the neuromuscular junction. May be seen as either repair of decrement or as an incremental response.
Pseudofacilitation	Occurs in normal muscle at high rates of stimulation as the muscles fire with improved synchrony, increasing amplitude but not area of the waveforms.
Safety factor	Refers to the amplitude above the threshold value needed to generate an action potential. In normal subjects this is due to an excessive release of acetylcholine in response to calcium uptake.

CMAP, compound muscle action potential.

Source: From American Association of Neuromuscular and Electrodiagnostic Medicine. Glossary of terms in neuromuscular electrodiagnostic medicine. *Muscle Nerve.* 2015;52:145–203. doi:10.1002/mus.24955

TABLE 28.2 Common Muscles Recorded for Repetitive Stimulation

Distal	Pros	Cons
• Ulnar to abductor digiti minimi • Median to abductor pollicis brevis • Fibular to tibialis anterior • Fibular to extensor digitorum brevis	• Less uncomfortable than proximal muscles • Easy to exercise to assess for increment • Commonly tested nerves making low initial compound muscle action potentials easy to recognize	• Less likely to show decrement in MG than proximal muscles
Midproximal		
• Spinal accessory to upper trapezius (posterior to sternocleidomastoid stimulation) • Axillary to deltoid (supraclavicular stimulation)	• Highly sensitive for decrement in MG	• Can be difficult to stabilize, but this is made easier in an upright individual by having him or her sit on the hands • Can be uncomfortable
Proximal		
• Facial to nasalis or orbicularis oculi (stylomastoid or preauricular stimulation)	• Most sensitive for decrement in MG	• Can be difficult to stabilize • Tend to get electrode movement with activation • Can be uncomfortable

MG, myasthenia gravis.

TABLE 28.3 Expected Findings in Pathologic Conditions

Postsynaptic Disorders—MG

Rule: Proximal muscles are generally more sensitive for finding decrement with slow stimulation in this condition.

Slow Stimulation	Postvoluntary Exercise/Fast Stimulation
• Motor studies should yield normal CMAP • MG is probable if decrement is >10% between the first and smallest of the next 4–5 responses on RS	• Increment can occur, but <40% • Can see postexercise exhaustion

Note: Partial or complete reversal of decrement after administration of anticholinesterase agents (e.g., edrophonium) generally confirms the diagnosis.

(continued)

TABLE 28.3 Expected Findings in Pathologic Conditions (*continued*)

Presynaptic Disorders—LEMS	
Rule: Distal muscles are as sensitive as proximal muscles, and generally easier to study for finding increment in this condition.	
Slow Stimulation	**Postvoluntary Exercise/Fast Stimulation**
• Motor studies are likely to yield a reduced CMAP • Decrement will frequently occur on RS in presynaptic disorders due to a reduced safety factor, but is not an essential diagnostic feature	• Postexercise facilitation with increment as high as 100%–200% can occur as the NMJ is flooded with acetylcholine during this technique • Postexercise exhaustion due to decreased excitability of the NMJ occurs 2–4 min after postexercise facilitation

Presynaptic Disorders—Botulism
Same as LEMS but increment with postexercise facilitation is not as dramatic and may not reach 100% *Note:* Lack of increment does not exclude botulism as a diagnosis.

CMAP, compound muscle action potential; LEMS, Lambert–Eaton myasthenic syndrome; MG, myasthenia gravis; NMJ, neuromuscular junction; RS, repetitive stimulation.

QUESTIONS

1. You are seeing a 56-year-old man with a history of type 1 diabetes mellitus controlled on an insulin pump referred to you for electrodiagnostic evaluation of weakness. He is a carpenter and reports that over the last 3 years it has been more difficult for him to hang cabinets. He denies any sensation changes. He has smoked one pack of tobacco cigarettes per day since the age of 18. He has difficulty getting out of his chair when moving to the examination table. On electrodiagnostic testing you would expect to see which of the following:

    A. Slowed conduction velocity in bilateral median motor studies
    B. An amplitude increase of greater than 100% in the postexercise phase on repetitive nerve stimulation
    C. Membrane instability in muscles innervated by cervical, thoracic, and lumbosacral spinal cord segments
    D. 10% decrement between the 1st and 7th stimulation in the baseline train of a repetitive nerve stimulation study
    E. Myopathic appearing motor units in the deltoid, biceps, and abductor pollicis brevis

---

Answers to the questions are located in Chapter 35.

2. You are consulted to perform an EMG on a patient in the intensive care unit who has acute-onset weakness and is now on a ventilator. The patient presented to the emergency department 18 hours prior when he thought he was having a stroke because he started to have blurry vision and slurred speech. These symptoms started in the evening; earlier in the day the patient was in his normal state of health and was able to attend a holiday picnic. On EMG you notice low compound muscle action potential (CMAP) amplitudes, a slight decrement on baseline repetitive nerve stimulation with about 30% increment on postexercise testing. The pathophysiology of this process is mediated by:
   A. Antibodies to the acetylcholine receptors on the postsynaptic membrane
   B. Antibodies to the voltage-gated calcium channels on the presynaptic membrane
   C. Toxin to the SNARE complex adhesion proteins preventing acetylcholine release
   D. An immune-mediated destruction of Schwann cell membranes

3. When setting up a study to evaluate suspected myasthenia gravis, which of the following is true?
   A. Repetitive nerve stimulation is often more sensitive when performed on proximal muscles rather than on distal muscles
   B. A study performed at cool temperatures is more likely to demonstrate a decremental response on repetitive nerve stimulation
   C. Single-fiber EMG is rarely helpful as it is uncommon to see increase jitter in myasthenia gravis
   D. High-frequency stimulation produces a more sensitive result than voluntary exercise for 1 minute and thus should always be done as part of repetitive nerve stimulation
   E. All of the above

ADDITIONAL READING

Keesey JC. AANEM minimonograph #33: electrodiagnostic approach to defects of neuromuscular transmission. *Muscle Nerve*. 1989;12:613–626. doi:10.1002/mus.880120802

Peripheral Neuropathy

Michael Mallow

INTRODUCTION

The electrodiagnostic evaluation of a patient with suspected peripheral neuropathy can be a daunting task for the budding consultant. The differential diagnosis is long and intimidating at first glance. The process, however, can be simplified if one applies precise technique, some basic principles of nerve physiology, and a systematic approach.

CLINICAL PRESENTATION

Patients will present with symptoms that are not confined to the distribution of one peripheral nerve or in the distribution of one nerve root. Commonly, symptoms will present in a length-dependent fashion. Sensory or motor symptoms may predominate depending on the nerves that are affected. The time course of symptoms should be obtained and will often provide insight into potential causes.

A complete motor and sensory examination should be performed in all patients presenting for electrodiagnostic evaluation of suspected peripheral neuropathy. Motor neuropathies may present with weakness or loss of muscle stretch reflexes, whereas sensory neuropathies often present with a "stocking-glove" distribution of sensory loss in the limbs. Any asymmetric abnormalities on examination should be noted and evaluated during electrodiagnostic testing.

Diabetic neuropathy affects nearly 50% of patients with the disease and is one of the most common causes of peripheral neuropathy. It is therefore frequently encountered in the EMG laboratory. Pathology is due to metabolic and vascular disruption of normal nerve conduction (1).

ELECTRODIAGNOSTIC APPROACH

Each electrodiagnostic examination should be tailored to the individual patient and, consequently, no one "protocol" is appropriate for every patient with suspected peripheral neuropathy. A suggested approach is provided here (2):

- Conduction studies:
  - Fibular and tibial motor studies with F-waves
    - If these are abnormal, proceed to ulnar and median motor studies.
  - Sural and median sensory studies

- Electromyography:
  - Tibialis anterior, gastrocnemius, first dorsal interosseous, and lumbar paraspinals
- Key points:
  - Abnormalities should prompt examination of the contralateral side.
  - Abnormalities suggestive of entrapment neuropathies must be thoroughly evaluated.
- Analyzing data:
  - The electromyographer is tasked with answering three questions when assessing a peripheral neuropathy:
    - ☐ Is the primary pathology axon loss or demyelination, or both?
    - ☐ Are motor or sensory nerves affected or are both affected?
    - ☐ Is the process diffuse or multifocal?
  - *Features of demyelination:* Demyelination has a conduction velocity less than 75% of normal and prolongation of distal latencies. Amplitudes may be normal but can be diminished in severe demyelination or in the setting of neuropraxia (conduction block). Needle EMG may show decreased recruitment.
  - *Features of axon loss:* Reduction in motor and sensory action potential amplitudes will be noted. Even the slowest axons conduct approximately 30 to 35 m/s. Lower conduction velocities indicate demyelination. Conduction velocity should not be less than 75% of normal. Needle EMG may show increased insertional activity and/or denervation potentials along with motor unit changes.

SUMMARY

The large differential diagnosis of peripheral neuropathy can be overwhelming early in training. Exhaustive lists of potential causes can be found in many texts. Commonly encountered diagnoses include:

Demyelinating
- Hereditary motor sensory neuropathy type 1
- Acute inflammatory demyelinating polyneuropathy (AIDP) or chronic inflammatory demyelinating polyneuropathy (CIDP)

Features of Demyelination and Axon Loss
- Diabetes
- Uremia

Axon Loss
- Alcohol
- Toxin exposure

QUESTIONS

1. Which of the following findings is most supportive of an axonal polyneuropathy?
    A. Prolongation of distal motor latencies
    B. Conduction block
    C. Low sensory amplitudes
    D. Prolongation of late responses

2. In acute inflammatory demyelinating polyneuropathy, which of the following is often the earliest finding on electrodiagnostic testing?
    A. Prolongation of late responses
    B. Motor amplitude loss
    C. Prolongation of distal sensory latencies
    D. Fibrillations on needle electromyography

3. If the peroneal motor nerve study recording at the extensor digitorum brevis does not elicit a response, what other muscle could be utilized?
    A. Tibialis anterior
    B. Medial gastrocnemius
    C. Abductor hallucis
    D. Abductor digiti minimi

REFERENCES

1. Pasnoor M, Dimachkie M, Kluding P, et al. Diabetic neuropathy part 1: overview and symmetric phenotypes. *Neurol Clin*. 2013;31(2):425–445. doi:10.1016/j.ncl.2013.02.004
2. Donofrio PD, Albers JW. AAEM minimonograph #34: polyneuropathy: classification by nerve conduction studies and electromyography. *Muscle Nerve*. 1990;13(10):889–903. doi:10.1002/mus.880131002

Answers to the questions are located in Chapter 35.

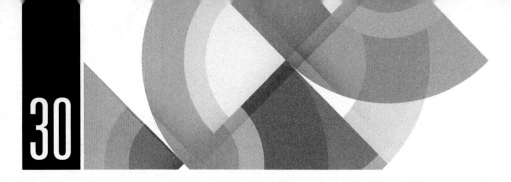

30

Brachial Plexopathy

Christopher J. Visco and Idris Amin

INTRODUCTION

Brachial plexopathy is one of the more challenging electrodiagnostic (EDX) diagnoses. The goals for an EDX evaluation include confirming that the patient indeed has a brachial plexopathy, determining which part of the plexus is affected, determining whether there is axonal involvement, and providing information to help determine the need for surgical intervention.

CLINICAL PRESENTATION

Limb and periscapular muscle weakness is the most common presentation of a person with a brachial plexopathy. Pain is a more variable symptom and is typically associated with trauma, neoplasm, and brachial neuritis. Postoperative plexopathies, rucksack-associated neuropathies, and radiation-induced neuropathies may present with minimal pain. In lower trunk injuries, patients may present with Horner syndrome (1).

- All evaluations should start with a thorough history followed by a complete neurological examination. Winging of the scapula may occur with brachial plexus lesions; the static and dynamic positions of the affected scapula may be associated with specific nerve lesions.
- The differential diagnosis of a patient presenting with upper limb pain and weakness is broad and includes other processes such as nerve root avulsions, radiculopathies, myelopathies, motor neuron disease, and peripheral nerve entrapments.

ANATOMY

The brachial plexus arises from five spinal nerve roots (C5–T1) and forms three trunks (upper, middle, and lower), six divisions (three anterior and three posterior), three cords (lateral, posterior, and medial), and five major terminal nerves (musculocutaneous, median, axillary, radial, and ulnar; Figure 30.1).

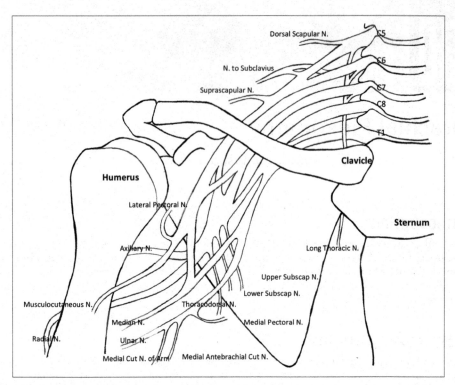

FIGURE 30.1 A graphical representation of the brachial plexus showing the roots, trunks, divisions, cords, and terminal nerves.
Source: Image courtesy of Susie Kwon, MD.

Classification

One common classification scheme for brachial plexopathies is based on anatomic location (Tables 30.1 and 30.2). This scheme divides brachial plexus injuries into two major anatomic categories: supraclavicular injuries (roots and trunks) versus infraclavicular injuries (cords and terminal nerves) (2). Other plexopathies do not have a site-specific predilection and are listed separately in Table 30.3 (3).

Anatomic Variants

There are many anatomic variants that can be seen in the brachial plexus. It is important to be familiar with some of the more common occurrences.

- Martin–Gruber anastomosis: Communicating nerve branch between the median nerve and ulnar nerve in the forearm; median motor nerve fibers cross over and innervate ulnar muscles; one study found Martin–Gruber anastomosis in 22.9% of cadavers (4)
- Median nerve formed by two lateral roots from lateral cord and one medial root from the medial cord (5,6)
- Long thoracic nerve pierces the middle scalene muscle (5,6)
- Lower trunk gives origin to the medial antebrachial cutaneous nerve (5)
- Suprascapular nerve originates directly from the C5 nerve root (5–7)

TABLE 30.1 Supraclavicular Injuries

Supraclavicular Injuries	Clinical Features	Electrodiagnostic Findings
Upper Plexus		
Burner syndrome	Abrupt, sharp, radiating upper limb pain associated with injuries in contact sports; symptoms usually temporary	If electrodiagnostic testing is ordered, it is often normal; may see some fibrillations in needle EMG of upper trunk muscles
Rucksack paralysis	Painless weakness following use of a rucksack or any type of backpack/harness	Associated with a demyelinating CB; sensory NCS normal; CB on motor NCS; Decreased recruitment pattern on needle EMG
Classic postoperative paralysis	Typically painless weakness associated with certain arm positions during the operation	Primarily demyelinating CB Sensory NCS normal; CB on motor NCS; decreased recruitment pattern on needle EMG
Lower Plexus		
Neurogenic TOS	Associated with a cervical rib; presents with C8/T1 weakness and thenar wasting, as well as paresthesias along the medial arm, forearm, and hand	SNAP abnormalities in medial antebrachial cutaneous nerve and ulnar to the 5th; abnormal median and ulnar motor; chronic axon loss noted in needle EMG of C8/T1 muscles
Postoperative TOS	Patient who had surgery for "disputed" TOS who, after surgery, developed brachial plexopathy	Findings are as listed for neurogenic TOS
Postmedian sternotomy plexopathy	Usually postcoronary artery bypass graft; related to traction or fractures of the first rib and primarily affects C8 and lower trunk	Needle EMG most useful in localizing lesion; need to differentiate from ulnar neuropathy
Pancoast syndrome	Refers to any lung disease (typically a tumor) that invades the lower trunk and C8/T1 roots; may be associated with Horner syndrome	NCS and needle EMG to help localize lesion

CB, conduction block; NCS, nerve conduction studies; SNAP, sensory nerve action potential; TOS, thoracic outlet syndrome.

TABLE 30.2 Typical Infraclavicular Injuries

Cords	Terminal Nerves
Lateral cord • Radiation (to the axillary lymph nodes)	Radial nerve • Crutch palsy Median nerve • Medial brachial fascial compartment syndrome
Medial cord • Midshaft clavicle fracture	Musculocutaneous • Surgical procedures performed near the coracoid process Axillary nerve • Glenohumeral dislocations • Proximal glenohumeral fractures

TABLE 30.3 Other Etiologies of Brachial Plexopathies

Etiology	Clinical Features	Electrodiagnostic Features
Neuralgic amyotrophy (Parsonage–Turner syndrome, brachial neuritis)	Abrupt severe shoulder pain, followed in 7–10 d by decreased pain and increased weakness	Tends to affect proximal motor nerves (long thoracic, suprascapular, and axillary)
Primary neoplastic (typically schwannomas and neurofibromas)	Painless mass followed by worsening paresthesias	More commonly affects sensory roots to the upper and middle plexus
Secondary neoplastic (due to extrinsic compression)	Associated with breast and lung cancers; severe shoulder and upper limb pain with weakness and paresthesias	Axillary node involvement typically affects medial cord and its branches
Radiation induced (most commonly related to breast cancer treatments)	Painless with paresthesias, followed by weakness	Tends to affect the lateral cord; look for myokymia on needle electromyography
Traumatic	Follows motor vehicle accident, sports, or work injuries	Electrodiagnostic results dependent on timing of tests

ELECTRODIAGNOSTIC APPROACH

Following the history and physical examination, the examiner, based on the formulated differential diagnosis, must be able to design an appropriate EDX study. A complete study involves studying both sensory and motor nerve conductions as well as a thorough needle EMG sampling, including the paraspinal musculature.

- Because most brachial plexopathies are considered a postganglionic process (excluding root avulsions), *sensory nerve action potential (SNAP)* amplitude abnormalities are very helpful in localizing the affected part of the plexus (Table 30.4). It is crucial to evaluate the SNAPs in both the affected and nonaffected limbs, as it is possible for SNAP amplitudes to be significantly diminished on the affected side but still within a normal range. Typically, if the SNAP amplitude of the affected side is less than 50% of the unaffected side, it is considered abnormal.
- Motor nerve conduction studies (NCS) can also be used to help localize lesions (Table 30.5). Similar to SNAPs, the *compound muscle action potential (CMAP)* values should be compared side to side to determine whether significant abnormalities exist. Motor nerves can be stimulated at multiple points, including proximal stimulation at the axilla and Erb point (Figure 30.2), to attempt to identify areas of conduction block.
- Needle EMG is then performed to further localize and confirm the lesion, based on the pattern of EMG abnormalities (Table 30.6). The EDX consultant should look for evidence of acute and ongoing denervation (fibrillations and positive sharp waves), chronic denervation (large amplitude, long duration, polyphasic motor units), and evidence of reduced neurogenic recruitment. Radiculopathy, in contrast to plexopathy, should have preserved SNAP amplitudes, positive paraspinal muscle abnormalities, and limb EMG abnormalities in a myotomal pattern.

TABLE 30.4 Typical Sensory Nerve Conduction Study Abnormalities in Brachial Plexopathies Based on Lesion Location

	Median to Thumb	Lateral Antebrachial Cutaneous Nerve	Superficial Radial	Median to Middle Finger	Ulnar to Little Finger	Medial Antebrachial Cutaneous Nerve
Upper trunk	■	■	■			
Middle trunk				■		
Lower trunk					■	■
Lateral cord	■	■		■		
Posterior cord			■			
Medial cord					■	■

NCS, nerve conduction study.
Note: Blackened cells indicate typical NCS abnormalities based on lesion location.

TABLE 30.5 Typical Motor Nerve Conduction Study Abnormalities in Brachial Plexopathies Based on Lesion Location

	Axillary to Deltoid	Musculocutaneous to Biceps	Radial to Extensor Digitorum Communis/ Extensor Indicis Proprius	Ulnar to Abductor Digiti Minimi/ First Dorsal Interossei	Median to Abductor Pollicis Brevis
Upper trunk	■	■	■		
Middle trunk			■		
Lower trunk			■	■	■
Lateral cord		■			■
Posterior cord	■		■		
Medial cord				■	■

NCS, nerve conduction study.

Note: Blackened cells indicate typical NCS abnormalities based on lesion location.

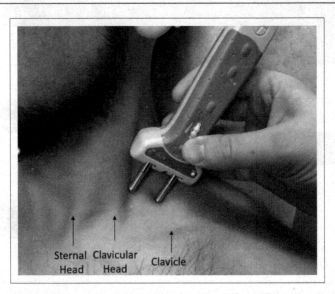

FIGURE 30.2 Illustration of the appropriate location for stimulation at Erb point. Note that stimulation occurs posterior to the clavicular head of the sternocleidomastoid muscle, and approximately 2 to 3 cm proximal to the clavicle.

TABLE 30.6 Typical Needle Electromyography Abnormalities in Brachial Plexopathies Based on Lesion Location

	Infraspinatus/ Supraspinatus	Deltoid	Bicep	Brachioradialis	Pronator Teres	Extensor Carpi Radialis Longus	Triceps	Flexor Carpi Radialis	Abductor Pollicis Brevis	Flexor Pollicis Longus	First Dorsal Interosseous	Flexor Carpi Ulnaris	Extensor Indicis Proprius
Upper trunk	●	●	●	●	●	●							
Middle trunk					●	●	●	●					●
Lower trunk									●	●	●	●	
Lateral cord			●		●			●					
Posterior cord		●		●		●	●						●
Medial cord									●	●	●	●	

Note: This chart represents the most common muscles involved in the various lesions and is not inclusive of all possible abnormalities. Blackened cells indicate typical abnormalities based on lesion location.

SUMMARY

Once brachial plexopathy is considered in the differential diagnosis, based on either the referral or the history and physical examination, the clinician must design a thorough study to determine whether brachial plexopathy or another neurological process is most likely responsible for the patient's symptoms and physical examination findings. At the end of the diagnostic study, the EDX consultant must then integrate the elements of the history, physical examination, and EDX study to arrive at a final impression.

QUESTIONS

1. A 44-year-old female presents to clinic with a 3-week history of severe right shoulder pain that started without any antecedent trauma. Pain is beginning to improve, but she is now noticing significant paresthesias and weakness lifting her arm. On examination, you notice some subtle winging of her right scapula, and weakness of arm abduction and external rotation. Needle EMG reveals fibrillations, positive sharp waves, and reduced recruitment in the serratus anterior, supraspinatus, and deltoid on the right with normal paraspinal muscles. Axillary compound muscle action potential amplitude also reduced significantly compared to unaffected side. The most likely diagnosis is:
   A. Radiculopathy based on the significant limb muscle needle EMG findings
   B. Rotator cuff injury with secondary muscle trauma causing needled EMG abnormalities
   C. Parsonage–Turner syndrome based on the classic history and predilection to affect certain nerves
   D. Unable to make diagnosis based on this information, MRI is needed

2. Which of the following statements regarding true neurogenic thoracic outlet syndrome is true?
   A. It primarily affects the upper trunk or lateral cord
   B. Abnormalities may be found in the ulnar sensory nerve action potential to fifth digit and the median and ulnar motor studies
   C. It would be common to find fibrillations and positive sharp waves in the biceps and deltoid
   D. Rarely do physical examination findings correlate with the electrodiagnostic findings

3. A 65-year-old female with a history of breast cancer with multiple treatments of radiation to her axillary lymph nodes, now presents with increasing paresthesias in her right upper limb and weakness in C8/T1 and lateral cord distribution without significant pain. Electrodiagnostic findings are consistent with lateral cord involvement with myokymia seen in needle EMG evaluation. Which of the following statements is true?
   A. The lack of significant pain is more consistent with a secondary neoplastic process
   B. The presence of myokymia and lateral cord involvement is most consistent with a radiation-induced cause
   C. The lack of complex repetitive discharges makes radiation-induced plexopathy unlikely
   D. Electrodiagnosis is of no value in this case and the patient should be referred for MRI

Answers to the questions are located in Chapter 35.

4. A 20-year-old male soldier presents with weakness of his left upper limb without significant pain shortly after carrying an 80-lb rucksack while deployed overseas. He denies any significant pain in the limb or shoulder. Which of the following statements is true?

   A. An x-ray should be obtained to evaluate for the presence of a cervical rib
   B. Electrodiagnostic studies will show evidence of a demyelinating conduction block
   C. This pathologic process is most likely due to an underlying autoimmune disorder
   D. There is likely an injury to an isolated peripheral nerve branch of the brachial plexus

REFERENCES

1. Sakellariou V, Badilas NK, Mazis GA, et al. Brachial plexus injuries in adults: evaluation and diagnostic approach. *ISRN Orthop*. 2014;2014:1–9. doi:10.1155/2014/726103
2. Dumitru D, Zwarts MJ. Brachial plexopathies and proximal mononeuropathies. In: Dumitru D, Amato AA, Zwarts MJ, eds. *Electrodiagnostic Medicine*. Philadelphia, PA: Hanley & Belfus; 2002:777–836.
3. Ferrante M. Brachial plexopathies: classification, causes, and consequences. *Muscle Nerve*. 2004;30:547–568. doi:10.1002/mus.20131
4. Rodriguez-Niedenführ M, Vazquez T, Parkin I, et al. Martin–Gruber anastomosis revisited. *Clin Anat*. 2002;15(2):129–134. doi:10.1002/ca.1107
5. Ememhadi M, Chabok SY, Samini F, et al. Anatomical variations of brachial plexus in adult cadavers: a descriptive study. *Arch Bone Jt Surg*. 2016;4(3):253–258. PubMed PMID: 27517072.
6. Fazan VPS, Amadeu AD, Caleffi AL, et al. Brachial plexus variations in its formation and main branches. *Acta Cir Bras*. 2003;18(suppl 5):14–18. doi:10.1590/S0102-86502003001200006
7. Tountas CP, Bergman RA. *Anatomic Variations of the Upper Extremity*. New York, NY: Churchill Livingstone; 1993.

31

Motor Neuron Disease

*Dena Abdelshahed, Ankita Dutta,
Chae K. Im, and James F. Wyss*

INTRODUCTION

Motor neuron diseases (MND) are a heterogenous group of inherited and acquired disorders caused by degeneration of motor neurons in the spinal cord, brainstem, and/or motor cortex. MND can affect upper motor neurons (UMN), lower motor neurons (LMN), or both (Table 31.1). The most famous and most common MND is amyotrophic lateral sclerosis (ALS), also known as *Lou Gehrig disease*, which affects both UMN and LMN. Lou Gehrig was a first baseman for the New York Yankees from 1923 to 1939 who played 2,130 consecutive games, earning him the nickname "The Iron Horse," and who famously delivered a retirement speech calling himself the "luckiest man on the face of this Earth" after being diagnosed with ALS. Primary lateral sclerosis (PLS) is an MND that is characterized only by UMN dysfunction, whereas progressive muscular atrophy (PMA) has only LMN dysfunction (Table 31.2). Many patients who are initially diagnosed with PLS or PMA eventually progress to ALS (1).

TABLE 31.1 Motor Neuron Diseases

UMN only: Primary lateral sclerosis
LMN only: Progressive muscular atrophy, spinal muscular atrophy, X-linked spinobulbar muscular atrophy (Kennedy disease)
Mixed UMN/LMN: Amyotrophic lateral sclerosis
Many atypical motor neuron diseases exist but are beyond the scope of this chapter.
LMN, lower motor neurons; UMN, upper motor neurons.

TABLE 31.2 Upper Motor Neuron Versus Lower Motor Neuron Signs

Upper motor neuron signs: Spastic weakness, spasticity, hyperreflexia, presence of a Hoffman and/or Babinski response
Lower motor neuron signs: Flaccid weakness, atrophy, hyporeflexia, and fasciculations

ANATOMY
Upper Motor Neuron

The UMN begins in the central nervous system and descends through the corticobulbar tract to the cranial nerve nuclei in the brainstem and through the corticospinal tract to the anterior horn cells in the spinal cord (Figure 31.1).

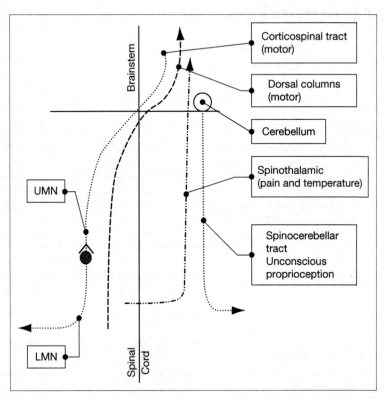

FIGURE 31.1 A schematic view of major long tracts in the spinal cord (ascending and descending arrows depict direction).

Lower Motor Neuron

The LMN includes the alpha motor neurons (Figure 31.2) that originate from the anterior horn cells in the gray matter of the spinal cord, and the cranial nerves that originate from nuclei in the brainstem.

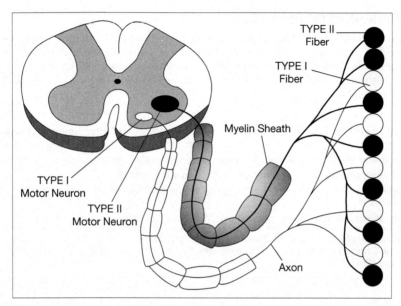

FIGURE 31.2 The motor unit. White and black represent type I and type II alpha motor neurons innervating multiple type I and type II muscle fibers, respectively.

Source: From Dumitru D. *Electrodiagnostic Medicine*. Philadelphia, PA: Hanley & Belfus; 1995, with permission.

CLINICAL PRESENTATION

Patients present with signs and symptoms related to UMN and/or LMN dysfunction (Table 31.2). Common complaints include weakness, cramping, stiffness, and functional decline. With bulbar dysfunction, complaints of sialorrhea, dysarthria, dysphagia, and eventually aspiration commonly occur. Cognition, sensation, and bowel/bladder function are typically spared.

The diagnosis of MND, including ALS, is made clinically and many experts use the revised El Escorial criteria to determine the probability of having ALS (1,2). Detailed history taking should aim to identify symptoms of UMN and/or LMN dysfunction. Physical examination is used to elicit UMN and/or LMN signs in all limbs and the bulbar region. Manual muscle testing will reveal weakness in the affected limbs and muscles, increased or decreased muscle stretch responses, and typically normal sensory testing. Additional diagnostic tests may include:

- Imaging modalities such as MRI of the cervical spine to rule out cervical cord pathology.
- Laboratory studies
  - Rule out treatable conditions such as vitamin B_{12} or folate deficiencies.
  - Perform superoxide dismutase testing (SOD1) to detect mutations in *SOD1* gene when a family history of MND is suspected.

ELECTRODIAGNOSTIC APPROACH

Although the diagnosis of MND is made clinically and not electrodiagnostically, electrodiagnostic (EDX) findings can support the diagnosis or help rule out alternate pathologies. Many experts use the revised El Escorial criteria, whereas others prefer Lambert's criteria for the EDX diagnosis of ALS (2,3). Please refer to Tables 31.3 and 31.4 for a recommended EDX protocol for MND (4).

TABLE 31.3 Recommended Nerve Conduction Study Protocol for Motor Neuron Disease

Routine motor studies for the median, ulnar, peroneal, and tibial nerves
Routine sensory studies for the median, ulnar, and sural nerves
Late responses should include F-waves for the median, ulnar, peroneal, and tibial nerves and H-reflexes
All of these studies should be performed on the more symptomatic side

Source: Adapted from Preston DC, Shapiro BE, eds. *Electromyography and Neuromuscular Disorders: Clinical-Electrophysiologic Correlations.* 2nd ed. Philadelphia, PA: Elsevier-Butterworth-Heinemann; 2005:428.

TABLE 31.4 Recommended Electromyographic Protocol for Motor Neuron Disease

At least three limbs should be sampled and the muscles chosen should be proximal and distal muscles with different peripheral nerve and root innervation
At least three segments of the thoracic paraspinals should be sampled, but avoid T11–12
At least one bulbar muscle (tongue, masseter, sternocleidomastoid, or facial muscles) should be sampled

Source: Adapted from Preston DC, Shapiro BE, eds. *Electromyography and Neuromuscular Disorders: Clinical-Electrophysiologic Correlations.* 2nd ed. Philadelphia, PA: Elsevier-Butterworth-Heinemann; 2005:431.

NERVE CONDUCTION STUDIES

Motor

- *Compound muscle action potential (CMAP)* amplitude is usually decreased due to axonal loss, but conduction velocity and latency may remain normal unless there has been significant loss of fast fiber axons.

Sensory

- *Sensory nerve action potential (SNAP)* amplitude, conduction velocity, and latency are classically expected to be normal; if these studies are abnormal, suspect an alternate or additional diagnosis. However, patients with Kennedy disease may have abnormal SNAPs.

Late Responses
- Responses are normal to slightly delayed depending on the amount of axon loss. This is a nonspecific finding as it may indicate pathology or dysfunction anywhere in the motor unit.

ELECTROMYOGRAPHY
This is the most important part of EDX testing in MND as it can detect LMN dysfunction before it becomes clinically apparent. To diagnose "definite" ALS, LMN abnormalities must be present in three different anatomic regions. Often, the most clinically involved muscles are tested first, but consideration should be made to test a variety of body regions, including thoracic paraspinals and/or accessory muscles of respiration as involvement of these regions increases the clinical suspicion of impending respiratory dysfunction (5).

Insertional Activity
- May be normal or increased.

Spontaneous Activity
- Fibrillation potentials and positive sharp waves (PSWs) will be present in involved muscles; fasciculations (e.g., ALS) or complex repetitive discharges (e.g., spinal muscular atrophy) may also be present.

Motor Unit Analysis
- Long duration, increased amplitude, and polyphasic motor unit action potentials (MUAPs) are typical.

Recruitment
- Reduced recruitment is a notable and common finding, with a reduced number of motor units firing at a rapid rate (5) (Table 31.5).

Repetitive Stimulation
- Collateral nerve terminal sprouting may lead to instability in neuromuscular transmission detected with single-fiber electromyography (EMG) or repetitive nerve stimulation (5).

OTHER DIAGNOSTIC TESTING
A recent study investigated the utility of MRI to aid in the diagnosis and monitoring of MND. Compared with healthy, age- and gender-matched controls, patients with MND had higher relative T2 muscle signals on a whole-body MRI. Higher T2 signal was associated with greater overall disability (6). On musculoskeletal ultrasound (MSK US), patients with MND have increased echogenicity within muscle and decreased muscle thickness. One study considered MSK US as a potential tool to monitor disease progression (7). More studies are needed to assess the clinical utility of diagnostic imaging in MND.

TABLE 31.5   Key Points

Motor neuron disease, especially amyotrophic lateral sclerosis, is a clinical diagnosis that should be supported by electrodiagnostic findings.
Physicians should look for signs of upper motor neuron and/or lower motor neuron dysfunction clinically and electrodiagnostically.
Many experts recommend testing at least three body regions that include the thoracic paraspinals and bulbar muscles.
Electromyography of the most affected muscles provides the highest yield of information.
Management is best provided by a specialized team of clinicians at neuromuscular clinics.

QUESTIONS

1. Which of the following is suggestive of lower motor neuron dysfunction?
    A. Spastic weakness
    B. Hyperreflexia
    C. Fasciculations
    D. Increased tone

2. Which of the following electrodiagnostic findings would lead you to question your diagnosis of motor neuron disease?
    A. Absence of positive sharp waves and fibrillation potentials in all tested muscles
    B. Decreased compound muscle action potential (CMAP) amplitudes
    C. Slightly delayed F-wave latency
    D. Normal CMAP conduction velocity

3. Which is true regarding motor unit recruitment in motor neuron disease (MND)?
    A. Motor unit recruitment is unaffected in MND and will be normal.
    B. Motor unit recruitment is reduced with an increased number of motor units firing at a slow rate.
    C. Motor unit recruitment is reduced with a reduced number of motor units firing at a rapid rate.
    D. Motor unit recruitment is reduced with a reduced number of motor units firing at a slow rate.

REFERENCES

1. Krivickas LS. Motor neuron disease. In: Frontera WR, Silver JK, Rizzo TD, eds. *Essentials of Physical Medicine and Rehabilitation*. 2nd ed. Philadelphia, PA: Saunders-Elsevier; 2008:705–712.
2. Brooks BR, Miller RG, Swash M, et al; World Federation of Neurology Research Group on Motor Neuron Diseases. El Escorial revisited: revised criteria for the diagnosis of amyotrophic lateral sclerosis. *Amyotroph Lateral Scler Other Motor Neuron Disord*. 2000;1: 293–299. PubMed PMID: 11464847.

Answers to the questions are located in Chapter 35.

3. Lambert E, Mulder D. Electromyographic studies in amyotrophic lateral sclerosis. *Proc Staff Meet Mayo Clin*. 1957;332:441–446. PubMed PMID: 13465824.
4. Preston DC, Shapiro BE. Amyotrophic lateral sclerosis and its variants. In: *Electromyography and Neuromuscular Disorders: Clinical-Electrophysiologic Correlations*. 2nd ed. Philadelphia, PA: Elsevier-Butterworth-Heinemann; 2005:423–437.
5. Joyce NC, Carter GT. Electrodiagnosis in persons with amyotrophic lateral sclerosis. *PM&R*. 2013;5(5 suppl):S89–S95. doi:10.1016/j.pmrj.2013.03.020
6. Jenkins TM, Alix JJP, David C, et al. Imaging muscle as a potential biomarker of denervation in motor neuron disease. *J Neurol Neurosurg Psychiatry*. 2018;89(3):248–255. doi:10.1136/jnnp-2017-316744
7. Shen J, Cartwright MS. Neuromuscular ultrasound in the assessment of polyneuropathies and motor neuron disease. *J Clin Neurophysiol*. 2016;33(2):86–93. doi:10.1097/WNP.0000000000000241

32

Myopathy

Gautam Malhotra

INTRODUCTION

A myopathy is any disease process in which the primary abnormality involves the muscle itself (rather than anterior horn cell, peripheral nerve, and neuromuscular junction). The inflammatory myopathies generally share common:

- Clinical features (acute or subacute onset, proximal symmetric muscle weakness, normal sensation, and normal to mildly diminished reflexes)
- Laboratory findings (elevated serum creatine kinase [CK], normal nerve conduction studies [NCS]).

Typical electromyographic findings include early recruitment of brief, small-amplitude, abundant polyphases (BSAPPs), and, in certain myopathies, membrane instability potentials. Muscle biopsy is ultimately used to identify the specific pathology.

CLINICAL PRESENTATION

The pertinent history and neuromuscular clinical examination findings are crucial in outlining the strategy for confirmatory studies (i.e., electrodiagnosis, biopsy, laboratory tests). The most common presenting symptom associated with myopathies is **weakness** that usually affects proximal musculature more than distal musculature (Table 32.1).

ELECTRODIAGNOSTIC APPROACH

Electrodiagnostic (EDX) testing is an extension of the history and physical examination to further evaluate the presentation of weakness. Other than myopathy, the common differential diagnosis must include disorders affecting the anterior horn cells, neuromuscular junction, radiculoplexopathies, demyelinating conditions, and so on. The EDX findings can direct further evaluations (e.g., muscle biopsy, imaging, genetic testing, and bloodwork).

TABLE 32.1 Some Key Findings of Clinical Presentation of Myopathies

Evaluation	Notable Presentations
Symptom: Weakness (reduced maximal force generation by a muscle group)	Distribution of weakness is of utmost importance. Commonly involves proximal symmetric limbs where weakness often presents with difficulty arising from a chair, negotiating stairs, or performing overhead activities. Severe or atypical cases can include weakness of the head, neck, and diaphragm. Some myopathies present with unusual patterns of weakness (e.g., scapulofibular, humerofibular, facioscapulohumeral).
Symptom: Other	Easy fatigability: Is unable to sustain a given level of force for a certain period. Nonspecific. Associated with repetitive activities. **Myalgia** or muscle pain is uncommon but may be seen in inflammatory myopathies. Sensory symptoms: Disorders other than myopathy should be suspected in the presence of paresthesias, although they may be subjective misperception of myalgias and muscle "twitching."
Other history	Developmental history, including motor milestones Family history and even examining affected family members Pediatric patients: Parents should be questioned with great care and sensitivity as they may unconsciously omit details or carry associated guilt.
Review of systems	Some medical problems are associated with specific myopathies (e.g., rashes, cardiac conduction problems, cataracts, and so on). Also look for indications of concomitant connective tissue diseases, metabolic conditions, endocrine disorders, toxicities, infection, or cancer.
Physical examination	Head: Difficulty whistling, frontal balding, temporal wasting, **head-drop** Limbs: Rashes, atrophy, **myotonia** (delayed relaxation or sustained contraction of muscle), paramyotonia (worsens with repetitive activity), **myoedema, Gower sign**, calf pseudohypertrophy, compensatory postures and movements, *scapular winging, trapezius hump* Neuro: Muscle stretch reflexes are initially preserved but progressively diminish and/or become unobtainable with profound loss of strength. Sensation should be normal in the setting of myopathy. If weakness is not obvious on manual muscle testing, look for difficulty with repetitive deep knee bending, climbing stairs, running, hopping on one foot, arising from a chair or floor, rising from a squat, repeated toe raises, and overhead arm raises against resistance. Gait evaluation may reveal lumbar hyperlordosis, waddling, **genu recurvatum**, wide-based stance, lurching, buckling, steppage, Trendelenburg sign, or foot-slap.

NERVE CONDUCTION STUDIES

- **Sensory nerve conduction studies:** *Sensory nerve action potential (SNAP)* amplitude, latency, and conduction velocity should all be within normal limits. The authors recommend testing one upper and one lower limb; if abnormalities are seen in SNAPs, then look for a peripheral nerve disorder. Reduced SNAP amplitudes can be encountered in elderly and edematous limbs and should be interpreted carefully. Conversely, abnormal SNAPs do not rule out myopathy, as it may be superimposed over a neuropathy.
- **Motor nerve conduction studies:** *Compound muscle action potential (CMAP)* distal motor latency and conduction velocity should be normal but amplitude may be diminished in damaged/involved muscle fibers. The authors recommend performing at least two motor studies in one upper and one lower limb. If CMAP amplitude is markedly diminished, one should rule out a presynaptic neuromuscular junction disorder (e.g., Lambert–Eaton and botulism) by obtaining CMAP after 10 seconds of isometric exercise (see Chapter 28). Typically, no increase from baseline will be seen with myopathy.
- **Late responses** (i.e., H-reflex, F-waves, blink reflexes) are also typically normal unless CMAP amplitudes are severely diminished. Of course, abnormal late responses may be seen in myopathy with concomitant demyelinating disorders (e.g., radiculopathy, demyelinating disease, entrapments, and so on).
- **Repetitive stimulation studies** can occasionally be abnormal in myopathies. When abnormal, every effort should be made to rule out an underlying peripheral nerve or neuromuscular junction disorder as well.

ELECTROMYOGRAPHY

- Insertional activity:
  - Experienced EDX consultant may note that the needle insertion "feels thin" (commonly encountered with corticosteroid-related myopathy) or "gritty" (i.e., varied resistance due to connective tissue replacement of muscle).
    - Normal **insertional activity** (i.e., brief burst of electrical activity with each needle motion) is typical with endocrine and chronic congenital myopathies.
    - Decreased or absent insertional activity can be encountered in fibrotic/fatty tissue.
    - *Increased* insertional activity in the form of runs of positive sharp waves, fibrillation potentials, and myotonic discharges can be seen in inflammatory and toxic myopathies.
  - **Abnormal sustained spontaneous activity:** Membrane instability potentials, such as complex repetitive discharges, positive sharp waves, and fibrillation potentials, may be encountered in many myopathies, especially inflammatory and toxic myopathies. Another common finding in myopathies is **myotonic discharges**, which are seen in channelopathies and dystrophies. During EMG, contracture may be encountered that manifests as electrical silence during muscle contraction.
- **Motor unit action potential (MUAP) morphology:** Remember BSAPP
  - **Brief:** Duration is the most consistent parameter for measurement in evaluating myopathy. The reduction is attributed to drop out of muscle fibers within the motor unit (MU).

- **Small amplitude:** Generally, myopathic MUAPs are low amplitude as a result of muscle damage and loss.
- **Polyphasic potentials:** They occur because of drop out of individual muscle fibers within the MU. There is increased variability in the size of myopathic muscle fibers, which results in an increased range of conduction velocities. This results in less synchronized summation of MUAP and manifests in increased serrations and phases.
- **Early recruitment:** Although the number of damaged fibers is variable, the number of MUs is unchanged before and after onset of myopathy (contrast with neuropathic picture). However, each MU generates less force than normal due to reduction in functioning muscle fibers per MU. The central nervous system (CNS) "sees" that insufficient force is being generated for the given number of activated MUs and recruits additional MUs at a frequency close to the onset frequency of the first MU. This phenomenon is known as **early recruitment**. It should be evoked with only a minimal amount of voluntary contraction. Keep in mind, recruitment testing with minimal voluntary effort usually evaluates type 1 fibers and may miss a myopathy affecting predominantly type 2 fibers.
- Distribution
  - Typically, myopathies present with proximal findings (common exceptions are inclusion body myositis and myotonic dystrophy). Check proximal muscles, including paraspinals, periscapular, glutei, and iliopsoas.
  - Information gleaned from needle EMG examination can be used to guide the surgeon in selecting the best muscle for biopsy. Needle examination should be limited to one side of the body while muscle biopsies are performed on the other. Unlike the biopsy, the needle EMG examination allows efficient evaluation of multiple muscles and multiple locations of each muscle.
- **Categorization:** The needle electromyographic examination may provide the most useful information about the properties of a patient's muscular tissue. A pattern of characteristic findings may suggest specific myopathic disease. Unfortunately, myopathies cannot be categorized by electrodiagnosis only:
  - A set of EDX findings are not pathognomonic of any one disease.
  - Multiple myopathies can have the same electrophysiologic presentation.
  - One myopathy can look different in different persons.

OTHER LABORATORY TESTING

- Electrolytes (especially calcium and potassium ions), thyroid/parathyroid function tests, erythrocyte sedimentation rate/antinuclear antibody, and enzymes (aspartate aminotransferase, lactate dehydrogenase, aldolase, gamma glutamyl transpeptidase)
- **CK is the most useful screening blood test:** Although CK level may be mildly elevated in rapidly degenerating neurogenic processes, it rarely exceeds 1,000 IU/L; keep in mind:
  - There is normal variability in CK levels depending on gender and race.
  - Not all myopathies have elevated serum CK levels.
  - CK levels do not correlate with degree of weakness in all patients.
  - CK levels are elevated after needle EMG, so avoid drawing CK levels for 2 to 3 days after needle EMG.

TABLE 32.2 A Suggested Classification of Myopathies

Noncongenital Muscular Dystrophies	Idiopathic Inflammatory Myopathies	Myopathies Associated With Systemic Disease	Nondystrophic Metabolic Myopathies	Nondystrophic Congenital Myopathies
• Duchenne • Becker • Emery–Dreifuss • Facioscapulohumeral • Limb girdle • Myotonic • Myoshi	• Dermatomyositis • Polymyositis • Inclusion body myositis • Necrotizing myositis	• HIV (*HIV-related inflammatory myopathy or AZT-related myopathy*) • Infections: *Viral, Trichinella, cysticercosis* • Thyroid disorders: *Hypothyroid or thyrotoxic myopathy* • Parathyroid disorders: *Hyperparathyroid or hypoparathyroid* • Corticosteroid atrophy and "steroid myopathy" • Sarcoidosis • Toxic myopathies: *ETOH, vincristine, chloroquine, AZT* • Electrolyte disturbance: *Low potassium, phosphorus, sodium, or calcium and high magnesium, calcium*	• Muscle phosphorylase deficiency • Type V glycogenosis, McArdle disease • Phosphofructokinase deficiency (type VII) • Acid maltase deficiency (type II) • Debranching enzyme deficiency (type III) • Carnitine deficiency	• Central core myopathy • Nemaline myopathy • Myotubular (centronuclear) myopathy • Congenital fiber type disproportion **Characterized by neonatal hypotonia or weakness; decreased spontaneous movement and delayed motor milestones, flabby muscles, high palate, pectus excavatum, elongated face, and scoliosis**

AZT, azidothymidine; ETOH, ethanol.

- Muscle biopsy
  - Choose a muscle that is mildly involved but not so severe that it may be impossible to distinguish myopathy from end-stage neurogenic damage.
  - CT/MRI or EDX may assist in muscle selection when there is no weakness; biopsy the muscles on the contralateral side to avoid the effect of syringomyositis (inflammatory changes due to EMG needle).
  - Open biopsy is a minor surgical procedure.
  - Normal muscle fibers are polygonal in shape with few inflammatory cells, with visible but not excessive amounts of connective tissue, and a characteristic checkerboard or mosaic pattern (Table 32.2).

QUESTIONS

1. Which of the following would not be classified as an idiopathic inflammatory myopathy?
   A. Dermatomyositis
   B. Polymyositis
   C. Inclusion body myositis
   D. Human immunodeficiency virus myositis

2. Which of the following is not a typical characteristic of motor unit action potentials observed during electromyography of patients with myopathy?
   A. Decreased (or delayed) recruitment
   B. Short duration
   C. Polyphasia
   D. Small amplitude

3. You perform electromyographic evaluation of a patient with new-onset proximal weakness, which reveals findings characteristic of an inflammatory myopathy. The degree of findings is as follows: left iliopsoas is severe, left vastus medialis is moderately severe, and left extensor hallucis is minimally involved. Which of the following is the best recommendation for muscle biopsy?
   A. Either left iliopsoas or right iliopsoas
   B. Right vastus medialis
   C. Left extensor hallucis
   D. Do not perform biopsy as it is of limited value in the workup of myopathies

4. Which of the following typically presents with proximal muscle weakness?
   A. Myotonic muscular dystrophy type 1
   B. Limb girdle muscular dystrophy
   C. Inclusion body myositis
   D. Polymyositis

Answers to the questions are located in Chapter 35.

The Use of Ultrasound With Electrodiagnosis

Jeffrey A. Strakowski

INTRODUCTION

High-frequency ultrasound is an excellent complimentary modality to electrodiagnostic techniques. It provides detailed anatomic correlation to the physiologic information obtained with electrodiagnosis. It has many advantages for assessing neuromuscular conditions over other imaging modalities. It can be used to assess pathology in peripheral nerves, mimicking neuromuscular conditions and muscles diseases. It can also be used to safely guide EMG needle insertion in vulnerable regions and assist with anatomic localization of challenging nerves and muscles.

ADVANTAGES OF USING ULTRASOUND WITH ELECTROPHYSIOLOGIC TECHNIQUES

- Provides anatomic correlation in focal neuropathies, and in some situations, the source.
- Can improve the precision of localization of focal neuropathies.
- Can typically provide useful information immediately after an acute neuropathy.
- Can be used to distinguish complete axonotmesis from neurotmesis (which is indistinguishable with electrodiagnosis).
- Is potentially more sensitive for detecting fasciculations.
- Can provide precise measurements of muscle and visualize muscle echotexture.
- Is not painful!

ADVANTAGES OF ULTRASOUND OVER OTHER IMAGING TECHNIQUES

- Is comparatively inexpensive.
- Uses no ionizing radiation and no known contraindications.
- Offers high resolution with better soft-tissue differentiation than conventional MRI.

- Can provide both a focused evaluation and an "on-the-spot" expanded evaluation.
- Allows easy side-to-side comparisons.
- Can provide dynamic assessment in real time.
- There are no problems with claustrophobia, pacemakers or other implants, or metallic foreign bodies.
- Can assess vascular flow.

PRINCIPLES OF IMAGING PERIPHERAL NERVES WITH ULTRASOUND
- Correctly identify the nerve tissue.
    - Do not confuse with neighboring vascular structures or tendons.
    - Nerves have a characteristic fascicular pattern (Figure 33.1).
- Use good technique and image optimization.
    - Use the highest frequency that allows sufficient penetration for best resolution.
    - Place the focal zone at the level of the structure of interest.
    - Set the depth so the structure of interest encompasses the majority of the screen.
    - Optimize the gain and gray-scale mapping for best contrast between nerve and surrounding tissue.
- Know the surrounding anatomy.
    - This helps with nerve identification as well as recognition of the influence of surrounding structures.
- Use consistent measurement techniques.
    - Cross-sectional area measurement in short axis is most commonly used and is most consistently reliable for identifying enlargement.
        - ☐ The transducer is placed perpendicular to the nerve for accuracy.
        - ☐ Measure the inner border of the outer epineurium (Figure 33.2).
- Assess the nerve in both short and long axis.
    - "One view is no view."
- Follow the course of the nerve.
    - Pathology can be missed if the inspection is isolated to small visual windows.

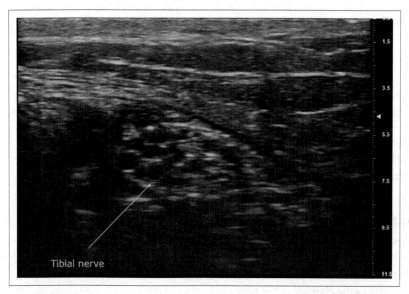

FIGURE 33.1 Sonogram demonstrating the fascicular pattern of the tibial nerve in short axis at the tarsal tunnel.

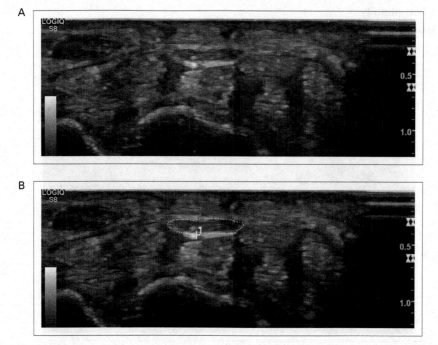

FIGURE 33.2 Sonograms demonstrating the median nerve at the carpal tunnel in short axis (A). Also shown is the technique for measuring the cross-sectional area of the nerve by performing a direct tracing at the inner border of the outer epineurium (B).

IMAGING STRATEGIES TO IMPROVE VISUALIZATION OF PERIPHERAL NERVES

- Use a liberal amount of coupling gel.
- More rapid and "back and forth" scanning will help distinguish nerve from other tissue.
- Use anatomic landmarks to help with localization.
- Pay attention to the degree of transducer pressure as this can affect the appearance of the tissue.
- Toggle and rock the transducer to create a perpendicular approach of the sound waves to minimize anisotropic artifact.
- Use Doppler flow to identify neighboring vascular structures.

SONOGRAPHIC FEATURES OF PERIPHERAL NERVE PATHOLOGY

- Abrupt changes in nerve caliper, including swelling or notching; use cross-sectional area and diameter measurement (Figure 33.3)
  - This can be seen with focal entrapments
- Irregularity in the contour of the nerve
- Irregularity or enlargement or loss of the nerve fascicles
  - This is often associated with axonal loss.
- Loss of continuity
  - Assess for neurotmesis in traumatic conditions.

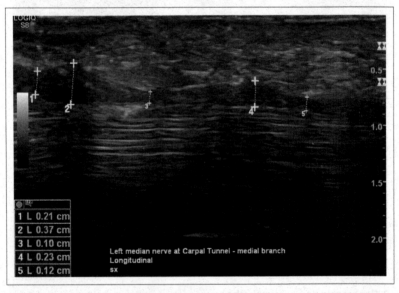

FIGURE 33.3 Sonogram demonstrating diameter measurement of a postsurgical median nerve at the carpal tunnel in long axis. In this view the extreme differences in caliper changes from the overlying hypertrophic scar are easily appreciated.

- Tumors or ganglia
- Relative vascularity
  - Generally, intraneural Doppler flow is not evident in normal peripheral nerves with conventional ultrasound.
- Abnormal mobility
  - This can be decreased with surrounding pressure or scarring and increased in some situations such as subluxation over bony prominences.
- Encroachment of surrounding tissue
  - Examples include fibrosis, compression, scarring, and encroaching muscles.

PRINCIPLES OF IMAGING MUSCLE FOR NEUROMUSCULAR ASSESSMENT WITH ULTRASOUND

- Inspect in more than one plane.
- Toggle the transducer to create optimum appearance.
  - Normal muscle is more hypoechoic than tendon and nerve.
- To inspect over a larger range, use somewhat lower frequency than imaging with peripheral nerve for larger muscles.
- Multiple focal zones should be used to create a more uniform appearance at different depths.
- Be familiar with the variety of muscle types and normal appearance.
- Assess muscles dynamically.
  - In long axis, they can be seen to lengthen with eccentric contraction and shorten with concentric contraction.

WHEN ASSESSING FOR NEUROMUSCULAR MUSCLE PATHOLOGY, INSPECT FOR:

- Muscle echotexture
  - Muscle becomes bright in pathologic conditions, such as denervation or myopathy, as a result of the loss of hypoechoic muscle fibers and the prominence of remaining connection tissue and fatty infiltration (Figure 33.4).
- Muscle size
  - Precise measurements can be obtained, including side-to-side differences in focal abnormalities.
- Pattern of abnormality
  - The muscle pattern of involvement can often provide valuable clues toward identifying a specific peripheral neuropathy or myopathy.
- Presence of trauma, strains, and herniations
- Fasciculations at rest

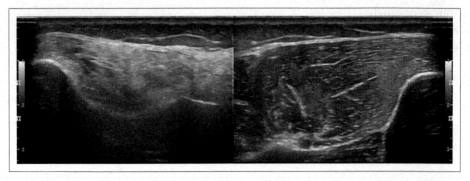

FIGURE 33.4 Sonogram demonstrating a side-to-side comparison of muscle appearance in the anterior compartment in an L5 radiculopathy. Note hyperechoic (bright) signal intensity and atrophy on the abnormal side (image on the left) relative to the normal muscle on the unaffected side (image on the right).

ULTRASOUND AS AN ADJUNCT TO ELECTRODIAGNOSTIC TECHNIQUES CAN BE USED

- As a teaching tool for peripheral nerve and muscle anatomy
- For improving accuracy for needle placement with electromyography (Figure 33.5)
- For improving safety with needle localizing in potentially vulnerable regions such as the diaphragm
- For assistance in localizing structures in anatomic variations and altered anatomy after surgery or trauma

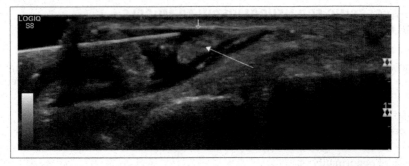

FIGURE 33.5 Sonogram demonstrating an in-plane visualization of the needle during a peripheral nerve (long white arrow) hydrodissection. Injectate is introduced around the nerve (short white arrow). The nerve is seen in short axis.

QUESTIONS

1. The most consistently reliable nerve measurement parameter for assessing a focal neuropathy on ultrasound is:
   A. Change in echotexture
   B. Enlargement of diameter in long axis
   C. Enlargement of the cross-sectional area in short axis
   D. The size of the refraction ratio

2. The hyperechoic signal at the outer portion of the nerve represents the:
   A. Epineurium
   B. Adventitial tissue
   C. Perineurium
   D. Intraneural fascicle

3. The advantage of a high-frequency transducer is:
   A. An increased footprint
   B. Better penetration
   C. Higher resolution of superficial structures
   D. Less flash artifact

4. The most effective way to reduce anisotropy of the tissue under examination is:
   A. Increase the gain
   B. Move the focal zone
   C. Toggle or rock the transducer to a more orthogonal position
   D. Decrease the depth

5. An advantage of ultrasound over electrophysiologic assessment in an acute traumatic nerve injury is that it can:
   A. Provide a better estimate of severity
   B. Provide a more specific indication of concomitant generalized nerve disease
   C. Distinguish complete axonotmesis from neurotmesis
   D. Distinguish complete axonotmesis from neurapraxia

ADDITIONAL READINGS

Bianchi S, Martinoli C. *Ultrasound of the Musculoskeletal System.* Heidelberg, Germany: Springer-Verlag; 2007.

Boon AJ, Oney-Marlow TM, Murphy NS, et al. Accuracy of electromyographic needle placement in cadavers: non-guided vs. ultrasound guided. *Muscle Nerve.* 2011;44(1):45–49. doi:10.1002/mus.22008

Answers to the questions are located in Chapter 35.

Peer S, Bodner G, eds. *High-Resolution Sonography of the Peripheral Nervous System*. 2nd ed. Berlin, Germany: Springer-Verlag; 2008.

Strakowski JA. *Ultrasound Evaluation of Focal Neuropathies. Correlation with Electrodiagnosis*. New York, NY: DemosMedical; 2014.

Strakowski JA. *Introduction to Musculoskeletal Ultrasound. Getting Started*. New York, NY: DemosMedical; 2016.

Tagliafico AS. Peripheral nerve imaging: Not only cross-sectional area. *World J Radiol*. 2016;8(8):726–728. doi:10.4329/wjr.v8.i8.726

Walker FO, Cartwright MS. *Neuromuscular Ultrasound*. Philadelphia, PA: Elsevier/Saunders; 2011.

Zaidman CM, van Alfen N. Ultrasound in the assessment of myopathic disorders. *J Clin Neurophysiol*. 2016;33(2):103–111. doi:10.1097/WNP.0000000000000245

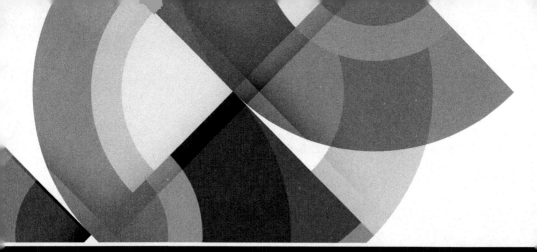

VI CHECKLISTS AND ANSWERS

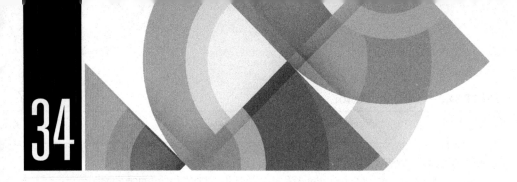

Checklists

UPPER LIMB MOTOR NERVE CONDUCTION STUDIES

TABLE 34.1 Ulnar Motor

Task
☐ Use the ADM muscle.
☐ Place the active electrode over the ADM muscle belly with the reference distal.
☐ Place the ground on the same limb.
☐ Measure 8 cm along the course of the ulnar nerve.
☐ Check to ensure the amplifier was on.
☐ Make sure the correct test was selected.
☐ Make sure the side (L/R) was correct.
☐ Start at a reasonable stimulation intensity.
☐ Set up the patient with the arm abducted and the elbow flexed.
☐ Stimulate at the wrist approximately near the FCU.
☐ Achieve supramaximal stimulation at the wrist.
☐ Stimulate approximately 3 cm distal to the ulnar groove.
☐ Achieve supramaximal stimulation at the elbow.
☐ Stimulate in the midarm.
☐ Achieve supramaximal stimulation at the midarm.
☐ Measure the distance from wrist to below elbow correctly.
☐ Measure the distance from below elbow to above elbow correctly.
ADM, abductor digiti minimi; FCU, flexor carpi ulnaris.

TABLE 34.2 Median Motor

Task
☐ Use the APB muscle.
☐ Place the active electrode over the APB muscle belly with the reference distal.
☐ Place the ground on the same limb.
☐ Measure 8 cm along the course of the median nerve.
☐ Check to ensure the amplifier was on.
☐ Make sure the correct test was selected.
☐ Make sure the side (L/R) was correct.
☐ Start at a reasonable stimulation intensity.
☐ Stimulate at the wrist approximately between the palmaris longus and FCR.
☐ Achieve supramaximal stimulation at the wrist.
☐ Stimulate medial to the biceps tendon.
☐ Achieve supramaximal stimulation medial to the biceps tendon.
☐ Measure the distance from the distal stimulation site to the proximal stimulation site correctly.

APB, abductor pollicis brevis; FCR, flexor carpi radialis.

UPPER LIMB SENSORY NERVE CONDUCTION STUDIES
TABLE 34.3 Median Sensory

Task
☐ Use the 2nd or 3rd digits.
☐ Use alcohol to prep the skin.
☐ Use the ring electrodes with the active proximal and the reference distal.
☐ Place the ground on the same limb between the active and the recording electrodes.
☐ Measure 14 cm along the course of the median nerve.
☐ Check to ensure the amplifier was on.
☐ Make sure the correct test was selected.
☐ Make sure the side (L/R) was correct.
☐ Start at a reasonable stimulation intensity.
☐ Stimulate at the wrist approximately between the palmaris longus and FCR.
☐ Achieve supramaximal stimulation.

FCR, flexor carpi radialis.

TABLE 34.4   Ulnar Sensory

Task
☐ Use the 5th digit.
☐ Use alcohol to prep the skin.
☐ Use the ring electrodes with the active proximal and the reference distal.
☐ Place the ground on the same limb between the active and the recording electrodes.
☐ Measure 14 cm along the course of the ulnar nerve.
☐ Check to ensure the amplifier was on.
☐ Make sure the correct test was selected.
☐ Make sure the side (L/R) was correct.
☐ Start at a reasonable stimulation intensity.
☐ Stimulate at the wrist approximately near the FCU.
☐ Achieve supramaximal stimulation.
FCU, flexor carpi ulnaris.

LOWER LIMB MOTOR NERVE CONDUCTION STUDIES
TABLE 34.5   Tibial Motor

Task
☐ Use the abductor hallucis muscle.
☐ Place the active electrode over the muscle belly of the abductor hallucis with the reference distal.
☐ Place the ground on the same limb.
☐ Measure 8 cm along the course of the tibial nerve.
☐ Check to ensure the amplifier was on.
☐ Make sure the correct test was selected.
☐ Make sure the side (L/R) was correct.
☐ Start at a reasonable stimulation intensity.
☐ Stimulate at the ankle approximately near the tendon of the tibialis anterior.
☐ Achieve supramaximal stimulation at the ankle.
☐ Stimulate just lateral to midline in the popliteal fossa.
☐ Achieve supramaximal stimulation at the popliteal fossa.
☐ Measure the distance from the ankle to the popliteal fossa correctly.

TABLE 34.6   Fibular Motor

Task
☐ Use the EDB muscle.
☐ Place the active electrode over the muscle belly of the EDB with the reference distal.
☐ Place the ground on the same limb.
☐ Measure 8 cm along the course of the fibular nerve.
☐ Check to ensure the amplifier was on.
☐ Make sure the correct test was selected.
☐ Make sure the side (L/R) was correct.
☐ Start at a reasonable stimulation intensity.
☐ Stimulate at the ankle approximately 1 cm posterior to the medial malleolus.
☐ Achieve supramaximal stimulation at the ankle.
☐ Stimulate at the lateral aspect of the popliteal fossa.
☐ Achieve supramaximal stimulation in the popliteal fossa.
☐ Measure the distance from the ankle to the popliteal fossa correctly.
EDB, extensor digitorum brevis.

LOWER LIMB SENSORY NERVE CONDUCTION STUDIES
TABLE 34.7   Sural Sensory

Task
☐ Use alcohol to prep the skin.
☐ Place bar electrode posterior to the lateral malleolus with the active proximal.
☐ Place the ground on the same limb between the active and the recording electrodes.
☐ Measure 14 cm along the course of the sural nerve.
☐ Check to ensure the amplifier was on.
☐ Make sure the correct test was selected.
☐ Make sure the side (L/R) was correct.
☐ Start at a reasonable stimulation intensity.
☐ Stimulate in the posterolateral leg.
☐ Achieve supramaximal stimulation.
☐ Troubleshoot appropriately if the waveform wasn't obtained initially.

DELAYED RESPONSES
TABLE 34.8 F-Wave

Task
☐ Correctly identify the muscle to be tested.
☐ Place the active electrode over the muscle belly with the reference distal.
☐ Place the ground on the same limb.
☐ Check to ensure the amplifier was on.
☐ Make sure the correct test was selected.
☐ Make sure the side (L/R) was correct.
☐ Start at a reasonable stimulation intensity.
☐ Stimulate at the appropriate distal stimulation site.
☐ Achieve supramaximal stimulation.
☐ Obtain at least 10 waveforms.
☐ Mark the minimal latency appropriately.

TABLE 34.9 H-Reflex

Task
☐ Use the soleus muscle.
☐ Measure from the popliteal fossa to the medial malleolus.
☐ Place the active electrode on the midpoint of a line between the popliteal fossa and the medial malleolus.
☐ Place the reference electrode on the Achilles tendon.
☐ Place the ground on the same limb.
☐ Check to ensure the amplifier was on.
☐ Make sure the correct test was selected.
☐ Make sure the side (L/R) was correct.
☐ Start at a low stimulation intensity.
☐ Stimulate just lateral to midline in the popliteal fossa.
☐ Increase the stimulation intensity appropriately to maximize the amplitude of the H-wave.
☐ Mark the minimal latency of the H-reflex appropriately.

ELECTROMYOGRAPHY
TABLE 34.10 Analysis of Spontaneous Activity

Task
☐ Use alcohol to prep the skin.
☐ Place the reference electrode on the muscle being tested relatively close to the location of the needle insertion.
☐ Place the ground on the same limb as the muscle being tested.
☐ Use appropriate gain and sensitivity for looking for spontaneous activity.
☐ Make the skin taut prior to entering the skin.
☐ Enter the skin with one short, quick motion.
☐ Check to ensure the amplifier was on and the amplitude was up.
☐ Evaluate five locations in one quadrant.
☐ Leave sufficient time between advancements to allow for evaluation.
☐ Withdraw the needle to just underneath the skin after finishing the first quadrant.
☐ Redirect the needle toward a 2nd quadrant.
☐ Evaluate four quadrants in the same manner.

RADICULOPATHY SCREENS
TABLE 34.11 Motor Unit Analysis and Recruitment

Task
☐ Change the gain and sweep speed to appropriately evaluate for motor unit analysis and recruitment.
☐ Ask the patient to activate the muscle with a low to moderate amount of resistance.
☐ Freeze the screen appropriately to analyze a motor unit and recruitment.
☐ Calculate the amplitude of a motor unit.
☐ Calculate the duration of a motor unit.
☐ State the number of phases of a motor unit.
☐ Calculate the firing rate of a motor unit.
☐ Ask the patient to activate the muscle with a maximal amount of resistance.
☐ Achieve an adequate interference pattern.
☐ Apply pressure with gauze if necessary after withdrawing the needle.
☐ Dispense the needle in a sharps container after completing the examination.

TABLE 34.12 Radiculopathy Screens

Cervical Radiculopathy Screen
Muscle
☐ Deltoid (axillary, C5–C6)
☐ Biceps (median, C5–C6)
☐ Triceps (radial, **C7**–C8–T1)
☐ Pronator teres (median, C6–C7)
☐ FDI (ulnar, C8–T1)
☐ APB (median, C8–T1)
Lumbar Radiculopathy Screen
Muscle
☐ Quadriceps (femoral, L2–**L3–L4**)
☐ Tibialis anterior (deep fibular, **L4–L5**)
☐ Peroneus longus (superficial fibular, **L5**–S1)
☐ Extensor hallucis longus (deep fibular, **L5**–S1)
☐ Tibialis posterior (tibial, L5–S1)
☐ Medial gastrocnemius (tibial, **S1**–S2)
APB, abductor pollicis brevis; FDI, first dorsal interosseous.

35

Answers to Multiple-Choice Questions

INSTRUMENTATION (Chapter 2)
1. C. Refer to the schematic. "Ground loop" and "signal processor" were distractors.
2. C. Refer to the schematic.
3. A. The differential amplifier subtracts the amplified signal of the second electrode from the first electrode. If the exact same current is entering both electrodes, they would cancel each other out and the resultant waveform would be a flatline.
4. C. The definition of a cathode is that it is a negatively charged electrode and cations are attracted to it. Option A is the opposite, in that the anode is positively charged and attracts anions. Options B and D are not defined by their charge. The ground electrode offers a reference point for the active (E1) and reference (E2) electrodes, whereas the reference electrode (E2) is used to subtract out noise common to the active electrode.
5. B. Gain is a unitless factor by which the input signal is amplified to get the output. Another explanation would be that gain is the ratio of output:input amplitudes. This is often confused with sensitivity (Option A), which is defined as the units per division on the screen (e.g., 1 mV per division). *Sweep* refers to the time per division on the *x*-axis. Option D is an attempt to misdirect toward a differential amplifier.

UPPER LIMB MOTOR STUDIES (Chapter 4)
1. E. All of the listed muscles are innervated by the ulnar nerve. Note that the ulnar nerve innervates all the intrinsic hand muscles EXCEPT for the LOAF muscles to the thumb and median half of the hand, which include lumbricals (lateral two), opponens pollicis, abductor pollicis brevis, and flexor pollicis brevis. A and D are incorrect because all of the muscles to the thumb are innervated by the median nerve, EXCEPT for adductor pollicis and deep head of flexor pollicis brevis, which are innervated by the ulnar nerve.
2. C. The ulnar nerve is tested in 90° shoulder abduction and elbow flexion; this places the nerve with as little slack as possible so that the distance measurements are more accurate.
3. B. The proximal stimulation site for the median motor nerve conduction study is at the antecubital fossa, medial to the biceps tendon. C is incorrect because the nerve is medial to the biceps tendon, not lateral. A is incorrect, this describes the distal stimulation site for the median nerve. D is incorrect, this describes the proximal stimulation site of the radial nerve.

4. B and D. The abductor pollicis brevis is innervated by the median nerve from levels C8–T1. The lower trunk and medial cord of the brachial plexus originate from the C8–T1 root levels. A and C are incorrect because the upper trunk arises from the C5–6 root levels and lateral cord arises from the anterior divisions of the C5–7 root levels. E is incorrect because the posterior cord contributes to the radial and axillary nerves.
5. B and D. The abductor digiti minimi is innervated by the ulnar nerve from levels C8–T1. The lower trunk and medial cord of the brachial plexus originate from the C8–T1 root levels. A, C, and E are incorrect as described in question 4.

UPPER LIMB SENSORY STUDIES (Chapter 5)

1. C. Decreasing the temperature results in both a delayed opening and a delayed closing of voltage-gated sodium and potassium channels. The delayed opening results in increased or delayed onset latency, therefore B and D are incorrect. The delayed closing results in more ions traversing the membrane and therefore a relatively larger amplitude, thereby making both A and B incorrect.
2. D. Known peripheral entrapments of the median nerve that could result in abnormal sensory nerve studies include both carpal tunnel syndrome and pronator teres entrapment syndrome. The medial cord of the brachial plexus makes contributions to both the ulnar and median nerves, and thus could result in abnormalities. Cervical radiculopathy can occur prior to the dorsal root ganglion, and thus have normal sensory nerve studies.
3. D. *Orthodromic studies* are defined as studies in which the stimulus travels the normal direction along the axon. *Antidromic studies* are defined as studies for which the direction is opposite of what is seen anatomically. Of the options listed, only the ulnar nerve transpalmar sensory with the distal stimulation and proximal recording describes the normal direction of sensory fiber conduction.
4. D. Multiple conditions can result in a delayed peak latency. Decreased temperature (option A) delays the opening of voltage-gated ion channels that can result in a delayed peak. Peripheral nerve entrapments such as carpal tunnel syndrome (option C) also can result in delayed peak. Stimulation over longer distances (option B) will also result in a delayed peak. Amyotrophic lateral sclerosis is a motor neuron disease and would have no effects on sensory nerve studies, making choice D correct.
5. B. The dorsal ulnar cutaneous (DUC) nerve is useful in differentiation. The DUC nerve is a sensory branch that leaves the main trunk on an average of 6 to 8 cm proximal to the ulnar styloid and becomes cutaneous as it passes between the flexor carpi ulnaris tendon and the ulna. It is therefore useful in localizing ulnar nerve lesions to the distal forearm or wrist, making option B correct.

LOWER LIMB MOTOR STUDIES (Chapter 6)

1. C. An accessory fibular nerve is the most common anomalous innervation in the lower extremity. It arises from the superficial fibular nerve and winds around the lateral malleolus, therefore stimulation should occur posterior to the lateral malleolus. A small compound muscle action potential (CMAP) will be evoked if an accessory fibular nerve is present. Option A is the stimulation point for the sural sensory study. Option B is the stimulation point for the superficial fibular sensory study. Option D is the stimulation point for the tibial motor study.

2. D. A popliteal cyst (or Baker's cyst) usually develops in the posteromedial popliteal fossa. Nerve compression may occur as the cyst grows in size and expands laterally. The tibial nerve is the most medial nerve of the neurovascular bundle in the popliteal fossa and is most likely affected. The sciatic nerve (option A) and common fibular nerve (option B) are rarely affected. The sural sensory nerve (option C) is not located in the popliteal fossa.
3. A. Failure to place the E1 electrode over the motor point during motor conduction studies will result in an initial positive deflection in the CMAP waveform. Options B, C, and D are incorrect because these will not result in an initial positive deflection.
4. D. The amplitude drop at the proximal stimulation (popliteal fossa) versus the distal (ankle) stimulation is greater with the tibial motor study than most other motor conduction studies. Normal controls may drop up to 50%. Therefore, a 40% drop is most likely within normal limits. Conduction block (option A) is much less likely; however, side-to-side comparisons may be useful if there is clinical suspicion for a conduction block involving the tibial nerve. Costimulation of the fibular nerve (option B) or an accessory tibial nerve (option C) would not cause an amplitude drop at the proximal stimulation.

LOWER LIMB SENSORY STUDIES (Chapter 7)

1. C. The sciatic nerve comprises a peroneal division that contributes to the superficial fibular (peroneal) nerve and the sural nerve, and a tibial division that contributes to the sural nerve. For this reason, an abnormality in both the superficial fibular (peroneal) sensory responses and sural responses could potentially localize to the sciatic nerve. A lesion of the common fibular (peroneal) nerve individually would not typically explain attenuated amplitudes in both sensory responses, the femoral nerve does not supply either the superficial fibular (peroneal) or sural nerves, nor does the lumbar plexus as the sciatic nerve comes off of the lumbosacral plexus.
2. C. The saphenous nerve takes off from the femoral nerve. Abnormal saphenous responses can be found in lumbar plexopathy, femoral neuropathy, isolated saphenous nerve injury, or peripheral neuropathy. Therefore, a lesion in the femoral nerve could explain both an abnormal femoral motor response and an abnormal saphenous response. The saphenous nerve is purely a sensory nerve, so an isolated saphenous abnormality would not explain both abnormalities (option A). A lesion proximal to the dorsal root ganglion as in a lumbar radiculopathy does not typically cause an abnormal sensory response, so the fact that the saphenous is impacted makes a radiculopathy much less likely (option B).
3. D. The lateral femoral cutaneous nerve is a pure sensory nerve formed from ventral divisions of L2/3 nerve roots, traveling through the lumbar plexus prior to its takeoff, where it then most commonly provides sensory innervation to the anterior lateral thigh. The lateral femoral cutaneous sensory response would not be expected to be abnormal in a radiculopathy (options A and B), as the lesion in a radiculopathy is typically proximal to the dorsal root ganglion. The lateral femoral cutaneous nerve does not travel with the femoral nerve, and so should be spared in a femoral neuropathy (option C).
4. C. The superficial fibular (peroneal) nerve may be abnormal in lesions of the lumbosacral plexus, sciatic nerve, common peroneal nerve, isolated superficial peroneal compressive neuropathies, peripheral neuropathies, and occasionally in L5 radiculopathies. Typically, the lateral femoral cutaneous, saphenous, and sural sensory responses are normal when a patient has a radiculopathy due to the location of the dorsal root ganglion in relation to common compression sites of the nerve root (options A, B, D).

5. B. The sural nerve is purely sensory and derived from the S1 nerve root (not L4) and is most often made up of two components: medial component from the tibial nerve and lateral component from the common peroneal nerve. In up to 25% of subjects, the sural nerve may be made up of components from the tibial or common peroneal nerves alone. As depicted in Figure 7.3, the sural nerve provides cutaneous innervation to the lateral portion of the leg and foot.
6. B. As depicted in Figure 7.7, the saphenous nerve provides cutaneous innervation to the medial aspect of the leg. The sural, superficial fibular (peroneal), and lateral femoral cutaneous nerves do not provide cutaneous innervation in the area of described numbness/paresthesia.

F-WAVES (Chapter 8)

1. B. The F-wave is only 1% to 5% the size of the respective compound muscle action potential (CMAP) because of the relatively small number of axons that are reactivated in the anterior horn. It may help to adjust the gain accordingly.
2. B. Ascending weakness is a hallmark of Guillain–Barré syndrome (GBS), which, as a presumptive diagnosis, would be appropriate to use F-wave studies as part of the electrodiagnostic (EDX) test.
3. A. The F-wave consists of afferent antidromic and efferent orthodromic motor.
4. D. When marking the minimal F-wave latency, the earliest F-wave is used. This is the fastest of any conduction on the rastered trace and theoretically should be representative of the largest fibers.
5. D. Meralgia paresthetica, or lateral femoral cutaneous neuropathy, is a condition affecting the lateral femoral cutaneous nerve, a cutaneous sensory nerve innervating the skin on the lateral part of the thigh. In conditions affecting the sensory nerves or nerve roots, F-waves are normal. Thus, F-wave studies would not be clinically relevant in assessing this condition. Options A, B, and C are all incorrect. Although F-waves have greater usefulness in detecting early polyradiculopathy (e.g., acute idiopathic demyelinating polyneuropathy [AIDP], GBS), they do maintain some value in assessing radiculopathy and polyneuropathy.
6. C. F-waves are entirely motor responses and do not have a synapse, therefore they would not be considered true reflexes. Option C describes the H-reflex. F-waves will vary with height, limb length, and age (option D). Each response will also vary in latency and amplitude depending on the size and speed of the conducting motor fiber (option B). F-waves may be present following submaximal stimulation, but are more pronounced after supramaximal stimulation with greater persistence and increased amplitude (option A).

H-REFLEXES (Chapter 9)

1. A. The H-reflex arc follows the same path in the tibial nerve as the Achilles reflex, afferent sensory (toward the cord), and efferent motor (away from the cord).
2. D. The latency can be prolonged when abnormal, but a normal study will have less than 2-ms difference from side to side. Because of the small margin of error, it is important to pay scrupulous attention to measuring and stimulating accurately on both limbs. The H-reflex is a submaximal stimulation and, as described in the chapter, can become smaller or disappear when approaching maximal or submaximal stimulation.
3. D. Any of the diagnoses listed could warrant the use of an H-reflex study depending on the circumstances and presentation, but it is most commonly used at the tibial nerve to the soleus evaluating for an S1 radiculopathy.

BASIC EMG TECHNIQUE (Chapter 10)

1. B. When a monopolar needle electrode is being used, a reference electrode is necessary. The reference should be near the location of needle insertion. If a concentric needle or single fiber needle is used, a separate reference electrode is not necessary because a reference is already built into the construction of concentric and single fiber needles. A ground electrode is needed for all studies.
2. C. There is no standard set number of muscles needed to examine in order to complete an electrodiagnostic study. Examining more muscles than is clinically necessary may cause excessive discomfort and risk to patients.
3. A. Needle advancements should be small, 1 mm or less, to minimize patient discomfort. Larger needle movements and sweeping needle movements cause more focal muscle trauma and therefore more discomfort.

BASIC APPROACH TO EMG WAVEFORM RECOGNITION (Chapter 11)

1. A. The other waveforms originate postjunctionally (i.e., at or distal to the endplate of the neuromuscular junction). Prejunctionally originating waveforms will not persist after experimentally blocking the neuromuscular junction.
2. B. Given similar duration, amplitude, morphology, and sonic character, trainees often confuse endplate spikes with fibrillation potentials. This is problematic as endplate spikes are normal spontaneous activity, whereas fibrillation potentials are considered abnormal. They can be discerned best by observing the rhythmicity (fibrillations are regular, whereas endplate spikes tend to be irregular) and morphology (fibrillations have initial deflections, whereas endplate spikes are usually the opposite). Options A and C are unlikely to be confused because of their typically larger amplitudes, durations, and morphology.
3. C. The other waveforms originate prejunctionally (i.e., somewhere along the neuron). Postjunctionally originating waveforms will persist even after neuromuscular blockade.
4. B. Fasciculation potentials are thought to be aberrantly originating somewhere along the motor neuron due to an unstable membrane. Myokymic discharges similarly begin along the neuronal membrane and may be ephaptically communicating with other neurons with poor membrane separation (possibly due to demyelination). Myotonic discharges are thought to be due to dysfunctional muscle membrane ion channels and not thought to transmit to other muscle membranes ephaptically.

MOTOR UNIT ACTION POTENTIAL ANALYSIS (Chapter 12)

1. D. A motor unit action potential (MUAP) duration correlates with the number of muscle fibers innervated by a single motor neuron in the region of the recording electrode. Option A is incorrect as the size of a MUAP is the summation of multiple muscle fibers. Option B is incorrect as the number of motor units supplying a muscle does not directly determine the size of each MUAP. Option C is incorrect, as the MUAP only represents summation of the muscle fiber action potentials of a particular motor unit that is within the recording area of the needle electrode.
2. D. The findings of increased amplitude, long duration, and polyphasicity are consistent with chronic denervation and reinnervation. Such long-duration, large-amplitude, and polyphasic MUAPs are characteristic for neuropathic process following collateral

reinnervation of previously denervated muscle fibers. Option A is incorrect as these MUAPs demonstrate findings outside the upper limit of normal for amplitude (generally, 6 mV for monopolar and 4 mV for concentric electrodes, respectively), increased duration (normal range 5–15 ms), and increased phasicity (normal range 2–4 phases). Option B is incorrect as MUAP size and shape do not usually change in the setting of acute or subacute axonal loss (up to 8 weeks). Option C is incorrect as the findings of increased amplitude, duration, and the number of phases are consistent with reinnervation.
3. E. Myopathic processes can cause short-duration, small-amplitude, and polyphasic MUAPs. Loss of muscle fiber integrity results in loss of muscle fiber action potential generation and hence leads to small-amplitude and short-duration MUAPs. Chronic myopathies, in which muscle fiber regeneration is occurring, can result in complex, polyphasic MUAPs. Occasionally, very chronic myopathies can result in long-duration MUAPs.
4. B. During axonal regeneration and sprouting (in contrast to collateral sprouting), early reinnervation will show small-amplitude and short-duration MUAPs. Option A is incorrect as Parsonage–Turner syndrome is a neuropathic condition and the findings of decreased recruitment would not be consistent with a myopathic condition (see Chapter 15). Options C and D are incorrect as a polyphasic motor unit related to collateral sprouting would result in increased duration of the MUAP.

RECRUITMENT (Chapter 13)

1. B. The firing rate of a motor unit action potential (MUAP) is calculated by determining how many times the MUAP is seen within a span of 1 second (e.g., if the sweep speed of the screen is set to 200 ms, multiply the number of MUAP occurrences by 5; if the sweep speed is set at 100 ms, multiply the number of MUAP occurrences by 10). Option A is incorrect because with a 4-Hz firing rate the MUAP would appear slightly less frequently than once every other sweep of the screen. Option C is incorrect as the MUAP would appear 10 times for each sweep of the screen. Option D is incorrect as the MUAP would appear 20 times on a single sweep of the screen.
2. C. Following a peripheral nerve injury that leads to axonal loss, reduced recruitment would be expected. Option A is incorrect as loss of axonal input to a muscle will result in reduced numbers of motor unit recruited (increase recruitment ratio). Option B is incorrect as increased (or "early") recruitment is expected in disorders affecting muscle rather than motor axons. Option D is incorrect as absent recruitment would only be expected in a nerve injury associated with complete axonal loss (conduction block in all motor axons).
3. C. Based on this screen sweep-speed setting, a single MUAP firing on each screen is consistent with 10 Hz (1 MUAP per 100 ms × 10 screens per second = 10 Hz). When an MUAP is firing greater than 10 Hz, the potential will move to the right on successive screens, and therefore 12 Hz is the correct answer. Option A is incorrect as an MUAP firing at less than 10 Hz would move to the left of the screen. Option B is incorrect as an MUAP would appear at the same position on the screen with each consecutive discharge. Option D is incorrect as an MUAP firing at 20 Hz would appear twice on each screen sweep.
4. C. An acute neuropathic process would result in axonal loss without signs of reinnervation. The term *picket fence appearance* has been used to describe reduced (discrete) MUAP recruitment. Option B is incorrect as delayed interference pattern would be unrelated to a neuropathic process and could support a central nervous system process. Option D is incorrect as an acute process would not allow time

for reinnervation (8 weeks or longer following injury), and therefore large and polyphasic MUAP would not be expected.

ORTHODROMIC AND ANTIDROMIC NERVE CONDUCTION STUDIES (Chapter 14)

1. A. The M-wave is the early response in the H-reflex, which represents direct transmission of the action potential from the stimulus distally toward the recording electrode. As the M-wave is the recording of a motor action potential, this is the physiologic direction of transmission and is, therefore, orthodromic. See Chapter 9 for more details of this study. Option B is not correct because this answer represents the opposite direction of transmission as described. Option C is not correct because this recording is a motor nerve conduction study. Option D is not correct because the M-wave is a physiologic response to the external stimulus provided.
2. B. An orthodromic sensory study does not stimulate motor nerve fibers and eliminates the motor nerve action potential signal in the recording. Option C is not correct because an antidromic sensory nerve study is typically performed by stimulation of a mixed-motor and sensory nerve and motor action potentials can be recorded. Option D is not correct because stimulation of a motor nerve will not avoid recording a motor action potential. Option A is not correct because the early and late efferent signal is a recording of the motor nerve action potential.
3. C. The action potential generated in both motor and sensory nerve conduction studies travels both distally and proximally. An example of this phenomenon is an F-wave, which produces early and late motor activation potentials. See Chapter 8 for further explanation of this study. Options A and B are not correct because the action potential travels both directions (ortho- and antidromic). Option D is not correct because the direction of the action potential is not temperature dependent.
4. C. The comparative studies for the combined sensory index (CSI) with stimulation proximally are antidromic and stimulation at the midpalm is orthodromic. See Chapter 5 for further explanation. Options A and B are not correct because the CSI is composed of multiple sensory studies, not motor. Option D is not correct because the CSI utilizes both anti- and orthodromic sensory studies.

TEMPORAL DISPERSION AND PHASE CANCELLATION (Chapter 15)

1. C. Temporal dispersion would be greatest for the sensory nerve action potential (SNAP) of the median nerve at the elbow. This is because temporal dispersion is most evident in sensory conductions rather than motor conductions, with a decrease in amplitude and increased duration seen with proximal compared to distal stimulation. Option A is not correct because distal stimulation is too close to the recording electrode to show increased temporal dispersion. Options B and D are not correct because temporal dispersion is most evident in sensory conductions.
2. B. Guillain–Barré syndrome or acute idiopathic demyelinating polyneuropathy (AIDP) classically demonstrates features of temporal dispersion and conduction block due to areas of focal demyelination along various nerves. Although option D (carpal tunnel syndrome) can show findings of demyelination across the wrist segment, temporal dispersion is most prevalent with longer nerve distances. Options A and C are incorrect. These are conditions that affect the anterior horn cell and neuromuscular junction, respectively. Temporal dispersion is not a major finding in those conditions.

3. **D.** In an acquired demyelinating neuropathy, it is common to see evidence of asymmetric, multifocal conduction block as well as temporal dispersion in addition to slowing of conduction. Options A and E are not correct. Uniform conduction velocity slowing is more likely seen with a hereditary demyelinating neuropathy such as Charcot–Marie–Tooth type I (HMSN type I).
4. **A.** Slight latency differences in SNAPs can cause the negative peaks of slower fibers to coincide with the positive peaks of faster fibers, leading up to a 50% reduction in SNAP area and amplitude. Option C is incorrect, because phase cancellation is most evident with longer distances where there is more time for separation and asynchronous firing of axon potentials. Options B and D are incorrect because less effect is noted with compound muscle action potentials (CMAPs) as they are of longer duration and less phase cancellation occurs as the potentials tend to superimpose more closely in phase over the same latency difference.
5. **F.** In this case, a better prognosis is suggested because distal motor amplitudes (wrist and below elbow) are within a normal range, whereas those above the elbow are reduced in amplitude, signifying a demyelinating lesion at the elbow. Options A, D, E, and G are incorrect. In an axonal lesion, distal amplitudes are also reduced in addition to reduced amplitude proximally, signifying loss of axons and a worse prognosis.

INTERPRETING STUDIES (Chapter 16)

1. **B.** It is recommended to wait 10 to 14 days after injury before performing nerve conduction studies. Motor and sensory axons may still remain excitable up to 7 to 10 days after injury, which may result in normal values if NCS is performed too early.
2. **A.** Axon loss will cause amplitude to be abnormal with stimulation both proximal and distal to the site of injury secondary to Wallerian degeneration. Options B and C are incorrect, as the amplitude loss with proximal stimulation must equal 20% or more to be defined as *conduction block*.
3. **B.** It typically takes 1 to 2 weeks for positive waves and fibrillations to develop in the paraspinals after a nerve injury and 3 to 6 weeks for paraspinals to develop in the limb muscles. It takes about 6 weeks for polyphasic potentials to be detectable after a nerve injury.
4. **D.** Motor units in myopathy are typically short duration, small amplitude, and polyphasic. Recruitment in myopathy is early or increased. Although insertional activity may show positive waves and fibrillations, especially in inflammatory myopathies, denervation also produces this finding. Normal electrodiagnostic findings are common in steroid myopathy, but normal findings would not help to confirm a diagnosis. Large-amplitude potentials with decreased recruitment are associated with chronic denervation.

COMMON ANOMALIES (Chapter 17)

1. **B.** The Martin–Gruber anastomosis (MGA) is an exchange where fibers that are destined to be part of the ulnar nerve at the wrist to innervate the first dorsal interosseous (FDI) instead initially travel with the median nerve, and then switch in the forearm. In someone without an MGA, normally both the ulnar wrist and elbow stimulation sites would contribute to the compound muscle action potential (CMAP) at the FDI. In an MGA, however, the fibers that are destined to supply the FDI travel along with the median nerve at the elbow and ulnar nerve at the wrist.

2. A. In an MGA, the fibers that are destined to supply the ulnar-innervated intrinsic hand muscles are traveling with the median nerve at the elbow, and therefore will be preserved if there is an ulnar nerve injury at the elbow. In both an ulnar-to-median crossover in the forearm and ulnar-to-median crossover in the hand (which is called a *Riche–Cannieu anomaly*), the ulnar intrinsic hand muscles would be affected, and the median nerve-innervated muscles may be affected as well.
3. D. To affect multiple C8–T1 muscles innervated by both the median (abductor pollicis brevis [APB]) and ulnar (abductor digiti minimi and FDI) nerves, one possibility is a Riche–Cannieu anomaly. However, the same pattern could be seen with a lower trunk injury or medial cord injury at the level of the brachial plexus. Either of those brachial plexus injuries can affect the medial antebrachial nerve, which would be spared in a Riche–Cannieu anomaly. Conversely, using a needle electrode (to minimize volume conduction) in the APB while stimulating the ulnar nerve would verify the presence of a Riche–Cannieu anomaly.
4. A. An anomalous innervation is often suspected when the amplitude at a proximal site (fibular head) is higher than at the distal site (ankle). The most common reason for this observation is understimulation at the distal site (ankle). Ensuring supramaximal stimulation at the distal site is very important in confirming an anomalous innervation. Option B is incorrect because it could lead to volume conduction and doesn't help ensure that the distal stimulation is optimized. Option C is incorrect because confirmation of an accessory fibular nerve would involve stimulation at the lateral malleolus. Option D is incorrect because option C is incorrect.

CARPAL TUNNEL SYNDROME (Chapter 18)

1. B. The anterior interosseous nerve braches off of the median nerve in the forearm and innervates pronator quadratus, flexor pollicis longus, and flexor digitorum to the 2nd and 3rd digits. Adductor pollicis and flexor digitorum profundus (FDP) to the 4th and 5th digits are innervated by the ulnar nerve. Extensor pollicis brevis is innervated by the radial nerve.
2. D. The table shows the three comparison studies used in the combined sensory index (CSI). All of the tests are based on the comparison between the median sensory nerve action potential (SNAP) peak latency to either the ulnar or radial SNAP peak latencies. Significant values for the transcarpal 8, median versus ulnar to digit IV, and median versus radial to digit I are >0.3 ms, >0.4 ms, and >0.5 ms, respectively. In this patient, the difference for the transcarpal 8 is significant (0.4 ms), but the median versus ulnar to digit IV (0.3 ms) and median versus radial to digit I (0.4 ms) are not significant for carpal tunnel syndrome (CTS). The CSI (the summation of the three individual studies) is 1.1, and a value greater than 0.9 ms indicates a diagnosis of CTS. The value of the CSI is that using all three studies in combination is more sensitive than using any of the studies independently.
3. A. If the median mononeuropathy is severe enough to cause atrophy, then the median motor study should be affected (abnormal), therefore option D is incorrect. If the nerve injury is severe enough to cause atrophy, then the motor response would show reduced amplitude due to axonal injury (correct answer is A). Options B and C show slowing in the median motor nerve only without axonal injury.
4. D. Electromyography is helpful to rule out other conditions that mimic carpal tunnel syndrome (options A and C) and can help describe the severity of the lesion (demyelinating versus axonal injury; option B). The correct answer is D, all of the above.

ULNAR NEUROPATHY AT THE ELBOW (Chapter 19)

1. **D.** Guyon's canal is a common area of compression of the ulnar nerve, particularly with cyclists who spend a great deal of time training (handlebar palsy). The ulnar nerve can get compressed in the flexor retinaculum causing sensory ailments such as numbness, tingling, or pain and, depending on the location, weakness of the intrinsic muscles of the hands. Options A and B are incorrect as these areas are not subject to compression during cycling activities as the wrist would be. Option C is incorrect as there are no areas of compression of the nerve in the midforearm.
2. **B.** Froment's sign is seen with weakness of the adductor pollicis, an ulnar nerve-innervated intrinsic muscle of the hand. The person is unable to adduct the thumb, thus the median nerve-innervated flexor pollicis longus is substituted. This results in thumb interphalangeal flexion to bring the thumb toward the index finger. Options A and C are incorrect as hyperextension of the metacarpophalangeal joints is seen with unopposed action of the extensor digitorum communis. This results in ulnar claw hand as the proximal interphalangeal (PIP) and distal interphalangeal (DIP) of the 4th and 5th digits subsequently remain in a flexed position due to weakness of the 3rd and 4th lumbricals. Option D is incorrect as the interossei adduct and abduct digits 2, 4, and 5 but not the thumb. Furthermore, the palmar cutaneous nerve only provides sensory innervation.
3. **C.** The flexor pollicis longus is innervated by the anterior interosseous nerve that branches from the median nerve, and thus would be normal with an ulnar neuropathy. The flexor digitor profundus (contribution to 4th and 5th digits), flexor digiti minimi, and first dorsal interossei are all innervated by the ulnar nerve.
4. **B.** The medial antebrachial cutaneous nerve branches directly from the medial cord. Option A is incorrect because the middle trunk of the brachial plexus does not contribute any divisions to the medial cord of the brachial plexus. The ulnar nerve does not supply the medial antebrachial cutaneous nerve, thus options C and D are incorrect.
5. **D.** The extensor indicis proprius is innervated by the radial nerve (roots C7, C8). Testing this muscle would help differentiate a C8 radiculopathy. Option A is incorrect as the pronator teres is innervated by the median nerve (roots C6, C7). Options B and C are incorrect as the flexor carpi ulnaris and palmaris brevis are both innervated by the ulnar nerve and therefore would not help in identifying a C8 radiculopathy.

RADIAL NEUROPATHY (Chapter 20)

1. **C.** The motor fibers of the posterior cord of the brachial plexus travel to the upper subscapular nerve (subscapularis innervation), lower subscapular nerve (subscapularis and teres major innervation), axillary nerve (deltoid and teres minor innervation), radial nerve, and the thoracodorsal nerve (latissimus dorsi innervation). Abnormal spontaneous activity on EMG in any of these peripheral nerve distributions should raise suspicion for a posterior cord lesion. Option A suggests a separate peripheral nerve, trunk level, or nerve root injury. Option B suggests cervical radiculopathy or another process. Option D would not help differentiate an isolated radial nerve injury.
2. **D.** Abnormal findings in the extensor carpi radialis longus increase the likelihood of a lesion above the lateral epicondyle. Normal findings in brachioradialis decrease the likelihood of a lesion at or above the spiral groove. Thus, a lesion occurring

below the spiral groove and above the lateral epicondyle is the most likely scenario.
3. B. Abnormal findings in the deltoid suggest a lesion proximal to the radial nerve and the level of the axilla. Normal findings in the triceps, brachioradialis, pronator teres, and cervical paraspinal muscles make nerve root involvement much less likely. A posterior cord lesion is the most likely scenario.
4. A. Abnormal findings in the cervical paraspinal muscles suggest a lesion at the level of the nerve roots or another process. Increased amplitude and duration and decreased recruitment in the affected muscles make myopathy less likely. Abnormal findings in the triceps, extensor carpi radialis longus, and flexor carpi ulnaris suggest a possible C7/C8 lesion, making nerve root involvement most likely.
5. D. Motor supply to the brachioradialis branches is inferior to the spiral groove and thus may exhibit abnormal spontaneous activity with electromyography after an injury at the spiral groove. The superficial radial nerve branches below the spiral groove and its action potential on nerve conduction study would likely be abnormal, especially in the setting of dorsal lateral hand numbness. The motor supply to anconeus branches above the spiral groove and would be unaffected. Extensor indicis proprius is supplied by the posterior interosseus nerve, which occurs below the spiral groove and would likely be affected in the presence of wrist drop.
6. C. Parsonage–Turner syndrome (also referred to as *brachial neuritis* and *neuralgic amyotrophy*) is an increasingly recognized source of posterior interosseus neuropathy and other peripheral mononeuropathies of the upper limb. A typical patient history may include initial onset of severe shoulder and upper extremity pain, which often occurs at night. As pain symptoms resolve, progressive weakness usually follows over days to weeks. On history, the patient may recall a period of flu-like illness preceding onset. Electrodiagnostic testing can be integral to help clarify the diagnosis along with MRI of the brachial plexus and peripheral nerves, which may demonstrate hourglass-like constrictions of the epineurium in the affected nerves.

ANTERIOR INTEROSSEOUS NERVE LESIONS (Chapter 21)

1. C. Patients with anterior interosseous nerve injuries will not be able to make an "OK" sign with their thumb and 2nd digit. Instead of the tips of their fingers touching, the volar surfaces of the fingers will be in contact secondary to the weakness of the flexor pollicis longus and the FDP muscles. Froment's sign and Wartenberg's sign are both characteristic of ulnar nerve injuries. The piano key sign is characteristic of radioulnar instability.
2. C. To isolate pronator quadratus muscle strength on physical examination, pronation should be tested when the elbow is flexed to reduce pronation from the pronator teres muscle.
3. D. Although the anterior interosseous nerve does provide sensory fibers to the wrist and interosseous membrane, there is no cutaneous innervation, so there should be no numbness.
4. B. A Martin–Gruber anastomosis is a median-to-ulnar crossover of fibers, and these fibers commonly are found in the anterior interosseous nerve. Thus, abnormalities may also be seen in the ulnar-innervated intrinsic muscles of the hand, such as the first dorsal interosseous muscle, adductor pollicis, and adductor digiti minimi.

FIBULAR (PERONEAL) NEUROPATHY (Chapter 22)

1. D. The answer is D because the deep fibular nerve innervates the sensory portion between the first and second digits. A, B, and C are incorrect because those sensory distributions are innervated mostly by the superficial fibular nerve.
2. D. In peroneal neuropathy, sensory changes consist of diminished sensation in the mid- and lower lateral calf as well as the dorsum of the foot between digits one and two. The lateral and plantar foot regions are usually spared. Motor changes consist of weakness in foot dorsiflexion and foot eversion. Option C is incorrect because the posterior tibial nerve that would be affected in tibial neuropathy allows for inversion and plantar flexion of the foot. These motor actions are preserved in peroneal neuropathy.
3. C. The answer is C, posterior to the lateral malleolus, because that is the path of the accessory fibular nerve. A, B, and D are incorrect as they are not proper locations for placements of electrodes.
4. C. Option C is correct because the sciatic nerve splits into the common fibular nerve and the tibial nerve just proximal to the posterior fossa. The common fibular nerve then innervates the short head of the biceps femoris and the lateral sensory aspect of the leg via the lateral cutaneous nerve before splitting into the deep and superficial branches. Option A's and B's group of muscles are innervated by the deep fibular nerve. Option C's group of muscles is innervated by the superficial fibular nerve.
5. B. Option B is correct because comparison to the unaffected limb must be made to see if abnormality in the affected limb is baseline. Options A, C, and D are not correct due to the incorrect limb and/or timing of study.
6. D. Option D is correct because ankle inversion is mostly done by the tibialis anterior, which is innervated by the posterior tibial nerve. Options A, B, and C are all done by muscles innervated by the common fibular nerve.

FEMORAL NEUROPATHY (Chapter 24)

1. A. Hunter's canal is also referred to as *adductor canal* or *subsartorial canal*; it is a fascial tunnel deep in the sartorius muscle along the anteromedial thigh. Inguinal ligament—the lateral femoral cutaneous nerve is often entrapped at this location. Posterior medial malleolus—the posterior tibial nerve is often entrapped at this location, in the tarsal tunnel. Extensor retinaculum of the ankle—the deep peroneal nerve can be entrapped at this location
2. D. L2, L3, and L4 paraspinals can help identify a radiculopathy at these levels. Rectus femoris is a femoral-innervated muscle. Adductor longus shares common nerve roots with the femoral nerve, but is innervated by the obturator nerve.
3. C. Abdominal or pelvic surgeries often can injure the femoral nerve due to lithotomy positioning or compression from retractors. The adductor longus muscle is innervated by the obturator nerve. The lateral surface of the thigh is innervated by the lateral femoral cutaneous nerve, which comes off of the lumbosacral plexus. A femoral neuropathy would result in a unilateral decrease in saphenous nerve action potentials, not bilateral.
4. B. Sensory nerve responses, such as the saphenous nerve, tend to be normal in radiculopathy, due to preferential injury to motor neurons from the disc. A lumbosacral plexopathy, saphenous mononeuropathy, and femoral mononeuropathy are all peripheral nerve injuries that would most likely affect motor and sensory fibers.

LUMBOSACRAL RADICULOPATHY (Chapter 25)

1. **B.** An EMG is an extension of your history and physical examination. It should be ordered when the diagnosis remains unclear. A test should only be ordered if it will affect your diagnosis, help with prognosis, or influence clinical decision-making. Option A is incorrect because although you may receive many referrals, ideally, you should make the clinical decision on whether the test is warranted. Option C is incorrect because you should treat the patient, not the image. Also, there is a high incidence of asymptomatic imaging abnormalities in the general population. Therefore, without a good history and physical examination, it is difficult to prove that the abnormality is the actual pain generator. If the history and examination correlated with the root level of the herniated disc, then, the diagnosis would already be clear and electrodiagnostic studies would most likely not be warranted. Option D is incorrect because the day of an injury is too early for most electrodiagnostic studies to show positive findings. Therefore, one might get a false negative reading. It is recommended to wait 3 weeks after the start of the symptoms in most cases. This is when fibrillation potentials and positive sharp waves will be seen in limb muscles.
2. **A.** Nerve root compression usually occurs proximal to the sensory dorsal root ganglion (DRG). The region of the nerve examined with the sensory nerve action potential (SNAP) techniques assesses only the fibers distal to the DRG that are still in contact with the healthy cell body. This statement describes the correct anatomical layout of the sensory nerve, region of pathology, and the correct region examined by SNAP techniques. Option B is incorrect because compression in a radiculopathy usually does not occur at, or distal to, the DRG. Option C is incorrect. Although this statement is true for the motor neuron, the sensory nerve cell body resides in the DRG. The question was referring to SNAPs, not compound muscle action potentials (CMAPs). Option D is incorrect because Wallerian degeneration will not occur distally if the DRG is still intact.
3. **D.** When paraspinal muscles are included as a part of the radiculopathy screen, a screen of six muscles (five limb plus paraspinals), representing all lumbosacral nerve root levels, will identify 98% to 100% of lumbosacral radiculopathies (option B). If paraspinal muscles cannot be reliably included, a screening of eight distal muscles should be used (option C). Thus, D is correct.

CERVICAL RADICULOPATHY (Chapter 26)

1. **A.** Weakness of right elbow extension is primarily from the triceps, which is a C6–7 innervated muscle. Weakness of wrist extension is from weak extensor carpi radialis (C6–7) and extensor carpi ulnaris (C7–8). Forearm pronation is controlled by pronator teres (C6–7) or pronator quadratus (C7–T1). Loss of triceps muscle stretch reflex on the right also indicates C7 spinal nerve involvement. The cervical spinal nerves exit above the level of the similarly numbered vertebrae, so the C7 spinal nerve exits near the C6–7 disc. Option B is incorrect because the symptoms do not correlate with disruption of the C6 spinal nerve. Options C and D are incorrect because there is no such thing as a C8 vertebra. There are only seven cervical vertebrae (C1–7).
2. **D.** This is not a C7 radiculopathy because the muscles with EMG abnormalities are all in the C7 myotome, but they do not have **different** peripheral nerve innervation. Triceps, extensor carpi radialis, and extensor carpi ulnaris (ECU) all receive peripheral innervation from the radial nerve. This is not a radial nerve mononeuropathy because nerve conduction studies (NCSs) were normal. Further testing is needed to clearly delineate whether this is a C7 radiculopathy and should start with a C7 muscle with different peripheral innervation: the pronator teres (C6–7, median nerve).

3. **C.** In consideration of mechanism of injury, cervical spinal radiculopathy and brachial plexus injury are possible diagnoses. Examination and EMG are consistent with possible C5 or C6 radiculopathy; however, an upper trunk brachial plexus injury may also present with these findings. Although plexus injury does not cause abnormal paraspinal EMG activity, test of this musculature (option A) will not be reliable amid tight posterior neck musculature. Another way to test for brachial plexus injury is to perform sensory NCS of a nerve with origin in the upper trunk of the brachial plexus (in this case, lateral antebrachial cutaneous [LAC]). NCS of LAC is expected to be abnormal in an upper trunk plexus injury and normal in a radiculopathy, in which the lesion is typically proximal to the dorsal root ganglion.
4. **B.** There is abnormal spontaneous activity in multiple muscles with C6 and C7 innervation, with normal testing of triceps brachii, which has C7 and C8 innervation, and normal deltoid, which also has C5 innervation. Overall, this test is consistent with C6 radiculopathy. This injury typically occurs at the root level, affecting the ventral portion, thus causing detriment to the efferent motor signal. In this injury, there is detriment to ventral rami, affecting appendicular musculature innervated through the brachial plexus, as well as to dorsal rami, affecting paraspinal musculature.
5. **C.** Abnormal activity within deltoid and biceps brachii on EMG does not distinguish a specific level of injury, as these muscles both have C5 and C6 innervation. In order to meet diagnostic criteria for a more specific root level, a C5-innervated muscle without C6 innervation and with different peripheral innervation could be tested. Rhomboids are C4 and C5 innervated, through the dorsal scapular nerve. Option B is incorrect, as paraspinal EMG will be unreliable with prior surgical instrumentation, and EMG of paraspinal musculature has low specificity for a single nerve root level.

FACIAL NERVE AND BLINK STUDIES (Chapter 27)
1. **C.** The active electrode (G1) is placed over the ipsilateral nasalis muscle in the facial motor NCS and, therefore, option D is incorrect. Options A and B are used for blink reflex study.
2. **C.** In trigeminal nerve lesions, ipsilateral R_1 and bilateral R_2 responses will be abnormal. In facial neuropathy, the R_1 and R_2 responses will be abnormal ipsilaterally and normal contralaterally and thus options A and B are incorrect. The chorda tympani nerve carries taste fibers to the anterior two thirds of the tongue and parasympathetic fibers to the salivary glands and thus option D is incorrect.
3. **A.** When the compound muscle action potential (CMAP) amplitude is less than 10% of that on the healthy side, maximum recovery will be delayed 6 to 12 months and function will be moderately or severely limited. If the amplitude is 10% to 30% of the healthy side, recovery may take 2 to 8 months with mild to moderate residua. If the CMAP amplitude is greater than 30% of normal, full complete recovery can be expected at 2 months after onset. Options B and C would be used to determine whether there is facial neuropathy but are not prognostic indicators. The CMAP amplitude between 5 and 7 days after injury is useful for prognosis and, therefore, option D is incorrect.
4. **B.** The blink reflex response (specifically, the R_2 response) on the side of a proximal facial nerve injury will be affected immediately. The facial motor nerve conduction study (option A) may be normal initially when the injury is proximal to the stimulation site, because axonal degeneration has not yet occurred. Similarly, needle EMG of the frontalis muscle (option C) may not show spontaneous activity when tested acutely, and also cannot be used to localize a proximal versus distal facial nerve lesion.

REPETITIVE STIMULATION AND NEUROMUSCULAR JUNCTION DISORDERS (Chapter 28)

1. **B.** Significant smoking history, type I diabetes mellitus, and generalized proximal weakness should raise concern for Lambert–Eaton myasthenic syndrome (LEMS), as it is commonly associated with small cell lung cancer and autoimmune disease. Electrodiagnostic testing in presynaptic disorders will reveal increment with postexercise facilitation. Motor nerve conduction studies will have decreased amplitudes but latencies and conduction velocities should not be affected. Needle EMG should have normal insertional activity and morphology. Although a decrement may be seen with slow repetitive stimulation, it should be seen between the first and fourth stimulation.
2. **C.** Foodborne illnesses are common after picnics, when proper food storage cannot occur. Sudden onset of bulbar symptoms is not likely to occur in myasthenia gravis (MG), which is associated with fatigable weakness. LEMS is rarely associated with bulbar symptoms as presenting symptoms.
3. **A.** Proximal muscles are more affected than distal muscles in MG. Cooler temperatures will improve decrement. Single fiber can be helpful in cases where repetitive stimulation is normal and will show increased jitter. High-frequency stimulation should be reserved only for patients who cannot perform exercise as it is quite painful.

PERIPHERAL NEUROPATHY (Chapter 29)

1. **C.** Loss of amplitude is a hallmark of axonal polyneuropathy.
2. **A.** F-wave and H-reflex abnormalities reflect the process of proximal demyelination seen in acute inflammatory demyelinating polyneuropathy.
3. **A.** Tibialis anterior is also innervated by the peroneal nerve more proximally.

BRACHIAL PLEXOPATHY (Chapter 30)

1. **C.** The history and physical describe the classic findings of Parsonage–Turner syndrome: proximal shoulder pain followed by weakness. The syndrome also shows a predilection for certain proximal nerves consistent with the electrodiagnostic (EDX) abnormalities shown earlier. Rotator cuff dysfunction would not show the EMG findings. A radiculopathy is unlikely based on the history and lack of paraspinal abnormalities. An MRI may be helpful in confirming diagnosis of Parsonage–Turner syndrome; it is not necessary in this case with classic history and EDX findings.
2. **B.** True neurogenic thoracic outlet syndrome (TOS) patients typically present with symptoms in the C8/T1 and lower trunk distribution. This should correlate to abnormalities of the ulnar sensory nerve action potential (SNAP) to the 5th digit and abnormalities to the median and ulnar motor. Needle abnormalities would be common in the first dorsal interosseous (FDI), not in the biceps or triceps. In true neurogenic TOS, the examination and electrodiagnostic findings typically correlate well.
3. **B.** Electrodiagnosis is very important to differentiate radiation-induced plexopathy from reoccurrence of cancer and should be used in conjunction with imaging. Lack of pain is more consistent with a radiation-induced cause. Radiation plexopathy tends to affect the lateral cord more frequently while secondary neoplastic processes favor the medial cord. Myokymia is associated with radiation-induced plexopathy.

4. B. Rucksack palsy is a brachial plexus lesion that is associated with wearing a heavy backpack on the shoulders. This is primarily a compressive lesion of the upper trunk of the brachial plexus. Electrodiagnostic studies in patients with rucksack palsy have been shown to demonstrate evidence of a demyelinating conduction block.

MOTOR NEURON DISEASE (Chapter 31)

1. C. Fasciculations, along with hyporeflexia, flaccid weakness, and atrophy are all lower motor neuron signs. Spastic weakness, spasticity, hyperreflexia, presence of a Hoffman and/or Babinski response are all upper motor neuron signs.
2. A. An absence of denervation potentials (i.e., fibrillations and positive sharp waves) in all tested muscles should cause you to question your diagnosis of a motor neuron disease because these will be present in involved muscles in a patient with motor neuron disease (MND). Decreased compound muscle action potential (CMAP) amplitude is consistent with the axon loss characteristic of MND. Delayed F-wave latency, although a nonspecific finding, may also be consistent with MND. In MND, CMAP conduction velocity will be preserved unless these is significant loss of fast fiber axons.
3. C. In MND, reduced motor unit recruitment is a notable and common finding with a reduced number of motor units firing at a rapid rate.

MYOPATHY (Chapter 32)

1. D. HIV is the cause so it is not idiopathic. The other three are classified as idiopathic inflammatory myopathies.
2. A. Typically myopathic motor unit action potential (MUAP) recruitment is increased or early.
3. C. Biopsy is very valuable in establishing the diagnosis of myopathy. Needle examination should be limited to one side of the body, whereas muscle biopsies are performed on the other. Recommend a muscle that is mildly involved but not so severe that it may be impossible to distinguish myopathy from end-stage neurogenic damage. In this case it would be the right vastus medialis.
4. D. The correct answer is polymyositis. The other answer choices are known for having distal presentations.

THE USE OF ULTRASOUND WITH ELECTRODIAGNOSIS (Chapter 33)

1. C. Cross-sectional area in short axis is the most consistently studied and used parameter for identifying enlargement in a focal neuropathy. Diameter in long axis is also helpful but more challenging to perform reliably and has been less studied. Change in echotexture is also important to distinguish but is generally less sensitive, particularly in milder or predominantly demyelinating lesions. Refraction ratio in not a measure for assessing peripheral nerve pathology.
2. A. The epineurium is the outer portion of the nerve that is generally hyperechoic relative to the internal darker nerve fascicles. The perineurium surrounds the individual nerve fascicles.
3. C. Higher frequency transducers provide better resolution but less penetration. The footprint with conventional linear transducers is a reflection of transducer size. Flash artifact occurs with movement with Doppler imaging.

4. C. Anisotropic artifact occurs with the incident beam of the sound waves not completely perpendicular to the structure of interest. This results in the signal reflecting away instead of back to the transducer, reducing clarity of the image. The alterations in the other answers will alter the image but not affect anisotropic artifact.
5. C. Electrophysiology can distinguish neuropraxia versus axonotmesis and is therefore a generally better measure of relative severity. It is also generally more effective in determining function in multiple nerves in a single assessment and is therefore often somewhat more reliable for helping diagnose many generalized neuromuscular conditions. Ultrasound can be used to effectively distinguish complete axonotmesis from neurotmesis, which are indistinguishable conditions with electrophysiology.

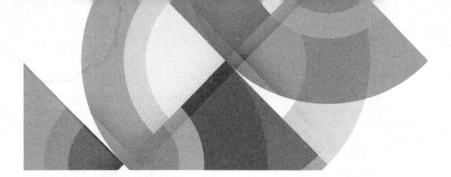

Index

abductor digiti minimi (ADM), 23–24, 28, 123, 141, 219
  anatomy, ulnar nerve, 137
  focal mononeuropathy, 112
  foot drop causes, 162
  inching technique, 139
  lead placement, 26
  lesion location, 226
  Martin–Gruber anastomosis, 155
  repetitive stimulation, 214
  routine nerve condition studies, 129
  ulnar neuropathy, frequently tested muscles, 140
abductor hallucis, 38
abductor pollicis brevis (APB)
  carpal tunnel, 128–129
  distal recording site, 24
  focal mononeuropathy, 112
  hand, median and motor nerves, 23
  lesion locations, 226
  Martin–Gruber anastomosis, 117–118
  needle EMG, 139–140
  repetitive stimulation, 214–215
  Riche–Cannieu anomaly, 119
  upper limb motor tests, 25
accessory fibular nerve (AFN)
  common anomalies, 116
  electrodiagnostic findings, 121
  functions, 121
  nerve conduction study, 122
  proximal stimulation, 164
action potentials (AP), 4, 11, 81, 103, 117
acute inflammatory demyelinating polyneuropathy (AIDP)
  demyelination, 218
  F-waves, 55
ADM. *See* abductor digiti minimi
AFN. *See* accessory fibular nerve
AIDP. *See* acute inflammatory demyelinating polyneuropathy

AIN. *See* anterior interosseous nerve
anomalies, common, 115–125
  technical errors, 115–116
anterior interosseous nerve (AIN), 116
  landmarks, 155
  lesions, 153–157
  Martin–Gruber anastomosis, 116
  muscle, 155
  pathophysiology, 153
anterior superior iliac spine (ASIS), 51–52, 179
antidromic median sensory nerve conduction study, 97–100
  electrode and stimulator placement, 98
  physiology, 97
AP. *See* action potentials
APB. *See* abductor pollicis brevis
area under the curve
  amplitude, 102
  race analogy, 102
arm/forearm
  posterior cutaneous nerve, 30
artifact management, 18
ASIS. *See* anterior superior iliac spine
axon loss
  amplitude, 108–109
  demyelination features, 218
axonal injury, 140. *See also* demyelinating injury; needle exam

Bactrian test, 130
Baker cyst, 170
biceps, 26–27, 160–161, 198, 200, 226, 261
  femoris, 44, 164, 170, 181
  tendon, 24–25, 139, 256
biopsy
  muscle selection, 242–243
  neuromuscular clinical examination, 239
black widow venom, 212

blink reflex study/blink studies, 203–209.
    See also facial nerve studies
  amplitude, 206
  late responses, 241
  nerve conduction studies, 205–206
  normal values, 207
botulism, 212, 215, 241
brachial plexopathies, 25, 154, 221–230
brachioradialis, 26–27, 143–144, 148–151, 195
brainstem, 6, 204, 231–232

calcium uptake, 213
carnitine deficiency, 243
carpal tunnel syndrome (CTS), 127–133
  cell carcinoma, 211
  distal nerve segments, 55
  EDX testing, 18
  Martin–Gruber anastomosis, 118
  median nerve, sensory branches, 30
  motor portion, 128
  Riche–Cannieu anomaly, 119
  sensory portion, 128
  Stevens criteria, 131
  upper limb motor test, 25
central nervous system, 56, 188, 232, 242
cervical radiculopathy, 195–201
  cervical spine cross section, 197
  classification, 222
  clinical symptom, 195
  electromyography muscle screen, 198, 261
  motor nerve conduction study, 197
  muscle testing, 198
  sensory nerve conduction study, 197
CMAPs. See compound muscle action potentials
CN. See cranial nerve
CNS. See central nervous system
combined sensory index (CSI), 29–30, 33, 98, 100, 129, 132
  median versus ulnar to digit IV test, 130
common nerve conduction study, 18
compound muscle action potentials (CMAPs)
  amplitude, 234
  brachial plexopathy, 225
  common anomalies, 115, 117–122
  EDX approach, 129, 154–155, 164, 212–213
  motor nerve conduction studies, 6, 188
  myopathy, 241
  phase cancellation, 101, 103–106
  sensory study, 18
  temporal dispersion, 101, 103–106
  waveform, 19
cranial nerve (CN), 203, 205, 232
CSI. See combined sensory index
CTS. See carpal tunnel syndrome

DABs. See dorsal abductors
demyelinating injury, features, 218
displays, 10–11
dorsal abductors (DABs), 24
dorsal root ganglion (DRG)
  lowerlimb sensory studies, 41
  neuropathic lesions, 109
  radiculopathy, 30, 186–188
  sensory nerve action potentials (SNAP), 97, 197
  spinal nerves, 196
dorsal ulnar cutaneous (DUC), 29–30, 32–34, 137–140
DRG. See dorsal root ganglion
DUC. See dorsal ulnar cutaneous

ECU. See extensor carpi ulnaris
EDB. See extensor digitorum brevis
EDC. See extensor digitorum communis
EDX. See electrodiagnostic
EIP. See extensor indicis proprius
elbow
  initial workup, 139
  ulnar neuropathy, 135–141
electrodes, 9
  recording and reference, 165
electrodiagnostic (EDX)
  accessory fibular nerve, 121
  basic principles, 3
  consult request, 4
  examination, 5
  history, 4
  instrumentation, 9–12
  logistical details, 3
  Martin–Gruber anastomosis, 118
  physical examination, 4
  sensory nerve conduction studies, 5
electromyography (EMG)
  abnormalities, diagnostic criteria, 197
  brachial plexopathies, lesion location, 227
  involuntary attributes, 7
  needle interpretation, 110–112
  single fiber, 213
  technique, 67–71
    procedure protocol, 69
  ulnar neuropathy, 140
evoked potentials, 6
evoked response, 5–6
  amplitiude, 5
  duration, 6, 82
extensor carpi ulnaris (ECU), 148, 275
extensor digitorum brevis (EDB)
  accessory fibular nerve, 121–122, 164–165
  EDX approach, 171

femoral neuropathy, 181
  lower limb motor studies, 37–39, 188
extensor digitorum communis (EDC),
    136, 143, 148
extensor indicis proprius (EIP), 25, 27
  radial neuropathy, 146–153
  ulnar neuropathy, 139–141

facial nerve studies, 203–209
facial neuropathy, 207
  lower motor neuron, 203
FCR. See flexor carpi radialis
FCU. See flexor carpi ulnaris
FDI. See first dorsal interosseous
FDP. See flexor digitorum profundus
FDS. See flexor digitorum superficialis
femoral neuropathy, 177–183
  electromyographic studies, 181–182
  motor nerve conduction studies, 180–181
  normal values, 180–181
fibrillation, positive sharp waves, 77
fibular motor, 258
  extensor to digitorum brevis, 37–38
fibular nerve, 39
fibular (peroneal) neuropathy, 159–167
firing rate, 89
first dorsal interosseous (FDI)
  Martin–Gruber anastomosis, 117–118
  ulnar neuropathy, elbow, 139–141
flexor carpi radialis (FCR), 32, 61, 112, 128
flexor carpi ulnaris (FCU)
  radial neuropathy, 143, 148–149
  ulnar nerve, 24
  ulnar neuropathy, elbow, 135, 137, 139–141
flexor digitorum profundus (FDP)
  anterior interosseous nerve lesion, 153–155
  carpal tunnel, 128
  ulnar neuropathy, elbow, 137–141
flexor digitorum superficialis (FDS), 128
flexor pollicis brevis (FPB), 28, 117
  carpal tunnel, 128
  deep head, 24
  superficial head, 23
  ulnar neuropathy, elbow, 137–138
flexor pollicis longus (FPL)
  anterior interosseous nerve lesion, 153–155
  carpal tunnel, 128
  ulnar neuropathy, elbow, 139, 141
foot drop, 161–163
FPB. See flexor pollicis brevis
FPL. See flexor pollicis longus
F-waves, 55–60, 197, 259
  amplitude, 57
  delayed responses, 175, 259
  Guillain–Barré syndrome, 56
  H-reflexes, comparison, 57
  late responses, 197
  limitations, 59

Guillain–Barré syndrome, 55–56, 61, 63
Guyon canal
  digital branches (after), 30
  dorsal ulnar cutaneous (before), 30

hand, median and ulnar muscles, 23
H-reflexes, 61, 198, 259
  amplitude, 57
  hypothenar eminence, 23
  late responses, 188–189
  setup, 62
  study performance, 62–63

indicis proprius, 147
infraclavicular injuries, 224
injury
  body's response to, 4
  sensory distributions, 138
  sites, tibial nerve entrapment or, 170
insertion activity, 74
interossei, 24
intrinsics, 23

junction
  distal myotendinous, 38
  musculotendinous, 44

knee extensors, 159, 177–178

latency, 16
lateral femoral cutaneous nerve
  conduction study, 51–52
  pathway and cutaneous distribution, 51–52
lesion
  location, brachial plexopathies, 225
  nerve conduction, 110
  neuropathic, 109
LMN. See lower motor neurons
lower limb motor nerve conduction studies, 37–40
  module 1 station 2, 257
  troubleshooting, 37–39
lower limb screen, 190
lower limb sensory studies, 41–54
lower motor neurons (LMN), 203, 231–232

lumbar radiculopathy screen, 261
lumbosacral radiculopathy, 185–193
lumbricals, 23

Martin–Gruber anastomosis (MGA), 122, 155–156, 222, 229
　comparison with hand anomalies, 116
　Marinacci anomaly, 119
　nerve conduction studies, 117–118
maximal stimulation, 15
membrane physiology, 4
MGA. *See* Martin–Gruber anastomosis
MND. *See* motor neuron diseases
motor nerve disease, latency, 5
motor neuron, spontaneous electrical activity, 74–76
motor neuron diseases (MND), 231–236, 277
　diagnostic testing, 235–236
　EDX testing, motor unit analysis, 235
　electromyographic protocol for, 234
　insertional activity, 235
　key points, 236
　late responses, 235
　lower motor neuron, 232
　nerve conduction study protocol for, 234
　sensory nerve action potential amplitude, 234
motor unit, amplitude, 111
motor unit action potential (MUAP)
　amplitude, 74, 82, 84
　characteristics and morphology in disease, 83
　denervation, 84
　duration, 82
　electromyography abnormalities, 198
　motor neuron disease, 235
　motor unit morphology, 82
　myopathies, 83, 241
　overview, 81
　reinnervation, 84
　stability, 83
MSR. *See* muscle stretch reflexes
MUAP. *See* motor unit action potential
muscle stretch reflexes (MSR), 185, 195, 199, 217, 240
myopathies, 239–244
　classification, 243
　key findings, 240
　lesions, 109

NCS. *See* nerve conduction studies
needle electromyography, 69–71
needle examination
　amplitude, 150–151
　anxiety and discomfort, reduction, 68
　axonal nerve injury, 112–113

nerve conduction studies (NCS), 3–4, 23–24, 28
　carpal tunnel syndrome, 131–132
　F-waves, 55–56
　femoral neuropathy, 179–183
　interpretation, limitations, 110
　lower limb motor, 258
　lower limb motor studies, 37–38
　lumbosacral radiculopathy, 187–188
　metrics, tibial nerve, 39
　phase cancellation, 102–104
　pregnancy, 17
　radial neuropathy, 146–147
　risks and contraindications for, 16–17
　systematic approach, 13–20
　temporal dispersion, 101–104
　ulnar neuropathy, elbow, 138–139
nerve stimulations, normal value range, 27, 33–34
normal value range, amplitude, 33–34, 180–181
neuromuscular system
　differential diagnosis, 18
　junction disorders, 211–216
　muscle pathology, 249–250

opponens digiti minimi, 23
opponens pollicis, 23
orthodromic conduction studies, 97–100
　physiology, 97
overstimulation, 15–16

pacemakers, defibrillators, 16
PACN. *See* posterior antebrachial cutaneous nerve
palmar adductors (PADs), 24
palmar branch (before carpal tunnel), 30
palmar ulnar cutaneous (before Guyon canal), 30
peripheral nerves
　imaging strategies, 248
　late responses, 6
　pathology, 248–249
peripheral neuropathy, 217–219
phase cancellation
　race analogy, 104
　temporal dispersion and, 104–105
phasicity, 83
pick-up electrodes, 6
PIN. *See* posterior interosseous nerve
positive sharp waves (PSW), 7, 75–78, 112, 141, 191, 198, 225, 228
posterior antebrachial cutaneous nerve (PACN), 149, 152
posterior interosseous nerve (PIN), 143–144, 146, 148
preshock checklist, 14

prestudy checklist, 13–14, 67–68
PSW. *See* positive sharp waves

quadriceps, 49, 180, 261

radial nerve, 25–26
 myotomes, 145
 sensory branches, 30
radial neuropathy, 143–152
 electrodiagnostic prognostic indicators, 149
 EMG screening in, 148
 nerve conduction studies, 146
 selected injuries, differential diagnosis, 148
 syndromes, 144
radiculopathy screens, 260–261
RCA. *See* Riche–Cannieu anomaly
recruitment
 analysis, 87
 assessment, 90
 clinical utility, 90
 maximal activation-interference pattern, 90
 myopathic processes, 92
 neuropathic processes, 91
 overview, 87
 quantitative parameters, 89
 ratio, 89
reference values, amplitude, 39
reflexes, components, 170
repetitive stimulation (RS), 211–215
 common muscles, 214
 definitions, 213
 pathologic conditions, 214–215
Riche–Cannieu anomaly (RCA), 116, 119–120, 122
 CTS nerve conduction study, 119
Robinson Index, 129–130
 median versus ulnar to digit IV test, 130
R_1 and R_2 responses, 207
RS. *See* repetitive stimulation

saphenous nerve
 pathway and cutaneous distribution, 48–50
 pelvis and upper thigh, 43
 study setup, 50
sciatic nerve, 37, 43
sensory nerve action potentials (SNAPs),
  5, 18, 41, 99
 carpal tunnel syndrome, 131–132
 lumbosacral radiculopathy, 187–188, 191–192
 physiologic nerve conductions, 97
 temporal dispersion and phase cancellation,
  101, 103
sensory placement, 99
signals, 10

SNAPs. *See* sensory nerve action potentials
spinal cord, 17
 long tracts, 232
spinal nerves, 43
spontaneous activity
 evaluation, 70
 module 1 station 4, 260
 waveform recognition, 75
stimulation, 25–27
 terminology, 15
stimulators, 11
 spinal cord and deep brain, 17
superficial fibular (peroneal) nerve
 pathway as well as cutaneous distribution, 46
 sensory conduction study, 147
 upper limb sensory, 30
superficial radial, 32–33
supraclavicular injuries, 223
sural nerve
 anatomy, 43–44
 conduction setup, 45
 cutaneous distribution, 44

temporal dispersion, 101
thenar eminence, 24
tibial
 motor
  abductor halluces, 38
  innervation, 170
  nerve conduction studies, 173
  study, trade secrets, 175–176
 nerve, sonogram, 247
 neuropathy, 169–176
 sensory innervation, 171
 sensory nerve condition studies, 172
  amplitude, 172–174
  lateral and medial plantar, 173–174
transcarpal 8 test, 130

ulnar nerve, 24
 abductor digiti minimi, 26
 anatomy, 137
 entrapment areas, 135
 little finger, 31, 33
 sensory branches, 30
 syndromes, 136
ulnar neuropathy, elbow, 135–141
 specific nerve conduction, 139
ultrasound
 electrodiagnostic techniques, 245–252
 imaging principles, 245–246
  neuromuscular assessment, 249
  peripheral nerves, 246

UMN. *See* upper motor neurons
upper limb motor nerve conduction studies, 23–28, 255–256
  checklists, 255–261
  lead placement, 25–27
  motor tests, 25–27
upper limb sensory, dorsal ulnar cutaneous, 32, 33
upper limb sensory studies, 29–34
upper motor neurons (UMN), 231–233
  versus lower motor neuron signs, 203–204, 231

visual displays, 10–11
volume conduction theory, 4
voluntary activity, 74
voluntary attributes, 7

waveform
  analysis, 17
  amplitude, 19–20
  checklists, 19–20
  CMAP, 19
  distal with proximal stimulation, 19